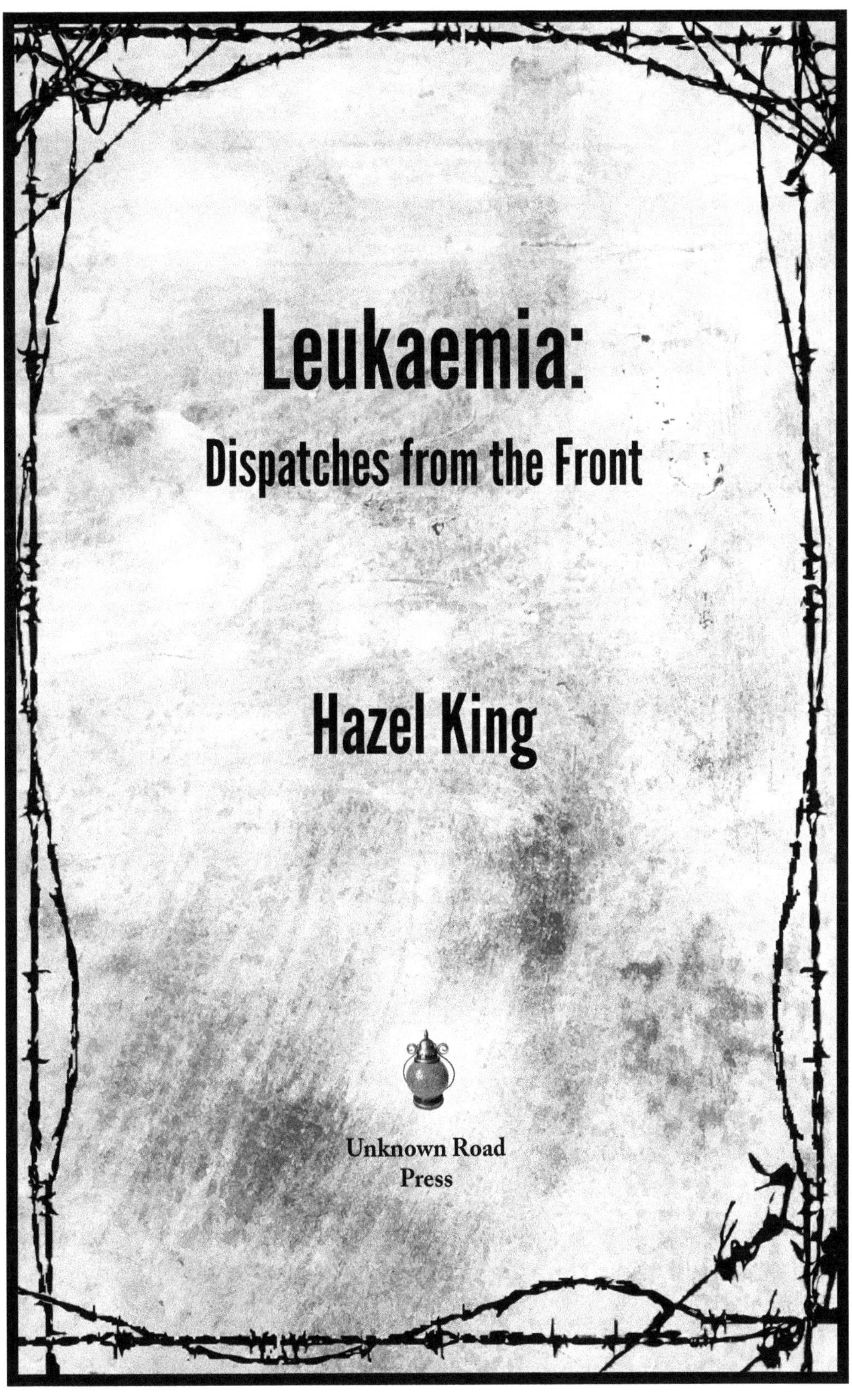

Leukaemia:

Dispatches from the Front

Hazel King

Unknown Road
Press

About the Author

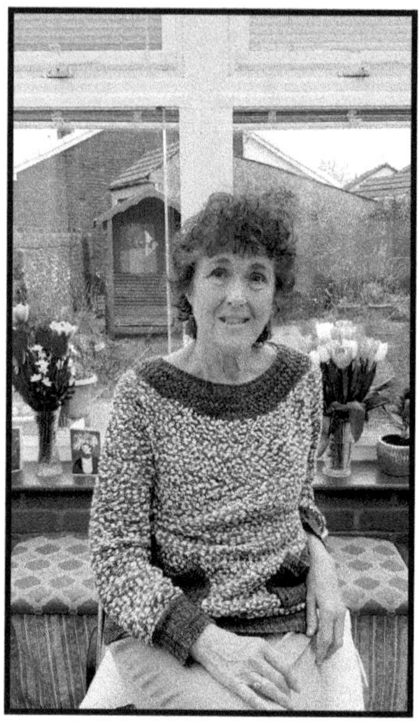

Hazel was born in the early 1950s in the South Wales Valleys into a coal mining family.

She has lived mostly in London – but spent a year in New York working with young ex-psychiatric patients; picked grapes in Israel and taught twice in the north of Nigeria.

She studied sociology at Reading University, and has an M.A. from the School of Oriental & African Studies in London. After her studies she had an article published in the *Journal of Religion in Africa* on the cooperation between two leaders, one Nigerian and the other Welsh, both well ahead of their times – and then decided to live her own life, while having the privilege at times of getting alongside others in their related research.

Having worked in shops, restaurants, and offices, it was unfortunately only teaching that enabled her to pay the mortgage. Later she started along with a musician, running music and dance workshops in primary schools, culminating in pupils deriving pride from showcasing their skills.

Now officially retired, she has been able to be a carer for her parents in Wales – one of the benefits of having survived a serious cancer, along with being able to add to her autobiography begun over a couple of decades ago! Indeed, this *Leukaemia: Dispatches from the Front*, will eventually form one of the chapters of a life lived in 5-year periods!

Her 'signature serious/humorous style' as it's been termed, is a dry humour from the valleys of her birth, but understood in certain cultures besides (others need training).

Email contact (unknownroadpress@gmail.com) is possible for feedback on the e-book, paperback or audio book, or to express interest in the eventual autobiography. She is not medically trained however, writing only of her own experience of AML Leukaemia, and so cannot offer advice which should be sought from a consultant.

Leukaemia: Dispatches from the Front

For information, e-mail:
unknownroadpress@gmail.com

First edition, 2021

ISBN 978-1-9168969-1-8

Dedicated to

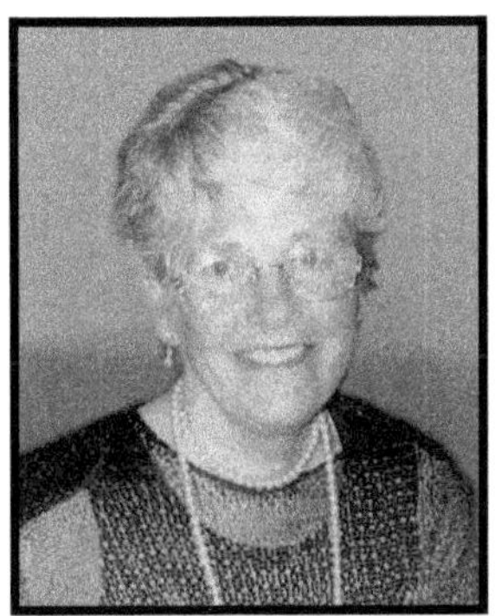

The memory of my friend Eileen
the best of people
who died in 2002 after Leukaemia.

A few years earlier, I had visited her in hospital with her son Michael Ronan.
It was Christmas Eve.
We were upset that she hadn't been given a diagnosis . . .
she *had* - but didn't want to spoil our Christmas.

Acknowledgements

With grateful thanks to the kind medics
of St Bartholomew's Hospital, London
particularly Prof Cavenagh, Dr Oakervee,
nurses & 'Dedicated Nurses'
(the cleaners & cooks too for they play their part);
family, especially my sister Jayne;
troops who prayed, sent cards & visited
– troopers Linda, & again Wendy,
even offering to look after me when discharged;
Deji (also Lawrence & Parnell) who helped with
the book format and proofreading;
the numerous blood donors & especially to my
bone marrow donor who chose to this day to remain
anonymous.
Not forgetting those who fought
to create & maintain the National Health Service
in the UK.

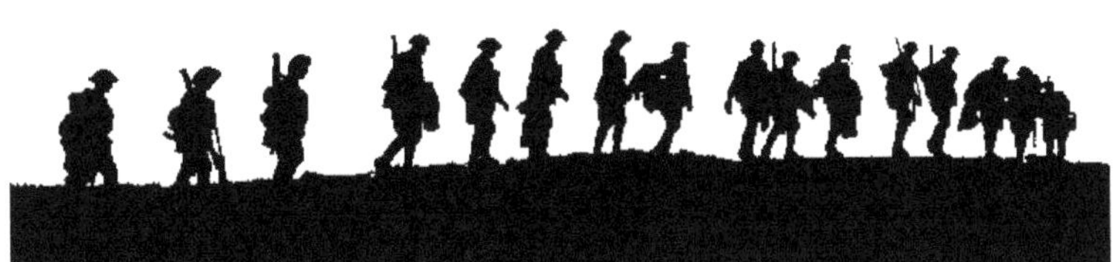

Plan of Engagement (aka Contents)

Lead-up to the Action

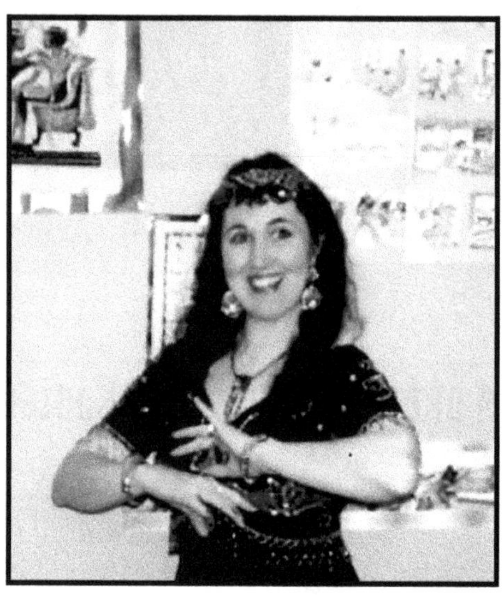

Day before admission – minding my own business running dance workshops in primary schools (publicity shot).

In the 6 days before volunteering myself at Accident & Emergency, I'd driven over 500 miles for work, and a friend's birthday house-party – all while feeling like 'death warmed up'. For over a year there'd been a strange, intermittent tiredness, unrelated to activity. Later I was told that I could have collapsed at any time 'including when you were driving'.

I wondered how they knew so quickly that I was desperately ill and sent a doctor out to find me before the blood sample had enough time to hit the lab – I came to learn that Leukaemia cells in later stages can form a visible film on the top. On hearing 'You'd better come back inside, we've had the first result', I was naively relieved – 'good, now they'll be able to cure me!'

I had known a neighbour, and also my friend's mother, who had had Leukaemia – it was something *other* people had. I had never associated it with myself, or indeed expected anything serious – thyroid perhaps!

Awaiting transfer, I was assigned a bed in a store cupboard: staff apologised as they came in for supplies, but it bothered me not at all – I was *in* the hospital, not *outside* it. However, something had to be done about the lack of rations – it was now night, nothing since breakfast and the canteen closed! I phoned my lodger to bring in my bananas, and then it also occurred to me that my friend Gurmiet lived a few blocks from the hospital and might have some left-over curry! Physical supplies secured, I rang another close friend for prayer cover over my shell-shocking news.

On being transferred to the main hospital late at night, no member of ward staff on duty was apparent. The ambulance men stood around, so I took charge and went looking for someone to enlist me.

Settled in my quarters and in the light of day, the thought occurred to me that there was a chance I could die. I looked online and saw age-wise I only had '*a chance*' of living. 'That can't be right!' I exclaimed, and decided not to look again. 'There is the chance of a cure', the Consultant said – and I thought I'd go with him!

I didn't accord with the 'Dedicated Nurse' I was assigned; I am not the touchy-feely type myself. I shared with my doctor that I was thinking of asking for a change. He listened and just said 'She's awfully good at her job'. Another choice made: Hazel would learn to adapt.

For 4 days I only informed folk on a need-to-know

basis that I was in hospital. I held back until the official diagnosis, so as not to have to sort out who'd been told what, if the initial 'we've seen Leukaemia cells', was incorrect.

My friend from Oxford where I'd rolled up the night before A&E (having failed to make it back to London in one go) suggested supporting me at the diagnosis meeting. Initial findings confirmed, there would be 3 rounds of chemo, the action to kick off in 2 days. I supposed somewhat dispassionately that I'd lose my hair. Viv queried whether a 'cold cap' could prevent hair loss. Not for this kind of chemo they dispassionately replied.

Without helmet then (and hoping head would not be lost along with hair), the request out for more uniforms (I had only 1 nightdress), battle lines decided, Generals & their Staff enlisted, I then began to write. The news blackout needed breaking with the first of my dispatches. It would come unannounced, and it would shock. Support may be needed *by them* I realised, and there was only me to give it; although my sister naturally took on that role for many of the folk in Wales, and those at church in London could support each other. Outside of these and workmates, was a group of friends spread across the globe largely known only to me.

I wrote as I observed almost like a war correspondent, some hardships of hospital being censored so as not to worry folk who could not help anyway: the nasty patient, who added unnecessary stress for me and for others, comes to mind (hey – you don't have to be nice to have Leukaemia); and the fact that although I had *lots* of visitors, none were regular enough to bring my few items of washing back, so I surreptitiously hung wet socks, etc. on a bar at the back of my cupboard and hoped no one would notice!

Medical information was completely unfamiliar to me, and I had to try passing it on to others. Someone into sci-fi might have understood the more fantastical elements through that lens. I was not. However, the war in Syria was all the news so a battle theme was very much in mind; and some of the complex issues, were understood through parallels with aspects of my faith.

So here are those email dispatches 'as sent' – with in the main just spellings and grammar improved. Most of the photos have been added for a wider audience (only a few of the photos were included at the time).

I'll end this chapter with a 1916 fun sketch of Barts' prep for another war – that against Zeppelin attack. The plan there, involved Guardsmen running through the courtyard garden with poles aloft, to hook through patients' mattress loops! The various wounded could count their blessings that they never actually had to be carried downstairs that way!

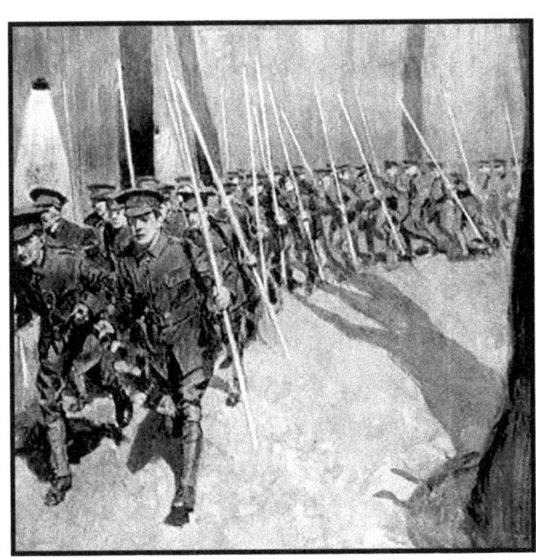

Dispatches sent:
October 2014 to October 2016

Friends 1

Dear Friends, Family, Church, & Music/Dance Colleagues,

You may wish to give yourself *time* to look at this email as I know it will make you all sad.

I'm sorry to tell you that I am *not at all well*. Last Thursday I was stubbornly performing in the Midlands, the next day I was at A&E. One woman in her time plays many parts!

A&E was not easy to impress with my various symptoms (one is reminded of Spike Milligan's epitaph on his grave 'See, I *told* you I was ill!') and the Dr said, 'Well you could have a blood test, it probably wouldn't show anything'.

Hazel said she would like – and was told to go home and ring in 2hrs for results. While looking around for a taxi, the Dr appeared outside the hospital looking around. Yes, he was looking for me as he'd seen the first result! & I was duly ushered in and later transferred to Barts (St Bartholomew's Hospital).

What I was told on re-entering the hospital has today been confirmed. I have Leukaemia. The common type. (Google can answer all your questions).

I will be here for a month for chemo to kill it all off – hopefully not the patient with it – after which the Phoenix may re-emerge.

Pause for you to take it in . . .

Practical points: my body will be engaged in a battle so

I'm going to be pretty busy & I do not have anyone to stand between me and all of you who care about me and genuinely want to know things, visit & help out.

So I plan to send intermittent email postings but you'd have to say you want to be on that list.

Important point: Lots of you will want to help but I will have no resistance to germs so kindly DO NOT CONTEMPLATE visiting if at all ill (5% of patients die of infections). Probably best to suggest a visit & wait for a reply. I have had 6 visitors in 4 days, as well as being terribly busy with procedures & my own business – so please don't think I'm lying here alone with no one to help. Also I will lose my hair, be sick & look it. Best to just get on with your own lives and see what transpires later – as Keats put it, to have:

the ability to dwell in uncertainty
without the restless desire to know.

How do I feel? At present I'm very philosophical about it all – my long-term future was sealed in a meeting in Reading Town Hall in 1971 – but naturally I would like not to precede my parents, and I would like to finish my autobiography, but these are out of my hands.

I'm in a top hospital – and along with that, your prayers, cards, and good wishes are all appreciated: Ward 4a, King George V Building, Barts Hosp, West Smithfields, London EC1A 7BE.

Don't be sad for long – go and do something nice for someone.

Regards,
Hazel

Friends 2

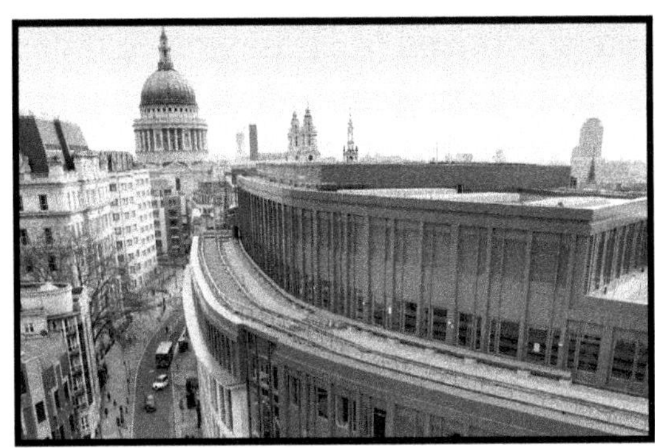

In the shadow of St Paul's Cathedral - St Bartholomew's Hospital.

Dear All who've asked to be on the list (plus 1 or 2 I'm sure just didn't heed instructions but could unsubscribe),

I hope you are all getting used to the news – I'm glad I haven't been as upset as some of you, but as you go on being taken up by the rest of life, I will from tomorrow morning be taken down to Point Zero by the start of chemo (by injection). Kill to cure. White blood cells in blood *all* have to go, can't discriminate – you didn't manage to sort them out yourself, so the American cavalry is coming, shoot on sight.

I'm prepared for the side effects – well I was until I saw how long the list was – but I possibly consider suffering the loss of fertility the worst (lol). Who knows my hair may grow back like my sister's – straight and blonde – but I rather suspect it will be one of the 50.

Had a visitor today but had to go off for a heart pulse after 10 min, you never know what's coming and when.

The good news is that my heart is strong enough for chemo. The bad news is that I have the heart of a 62-year-old woman (thought it might have matched the outside).

The ward of 4 women I am in (had a bit of time to talk to them today, yesterday too busy with emails, etc.) is now closed for 3 days in terms of us leaving (didn't seem to stop me going for the heart scan – I suppose they just don't want us fraternising with the other patients). *One of us* has a cold they announced! Elizabeth from Southern Sudan in bed opposite today 'fessed up that *she* had thought she was starting a cold following an Orderly sneezing in here. However, turns out she isn't, so don't know if that changes anything. It's a cross between *Prisoners of Cell Block H* and *Passport to Pimlico*.

A nice nearby friend wanted to visit tonight but I postponed her to another day as I'm really tired now.

Last night my jaw on one side started swelling & the difference in my face is very apparent. I reminded the very kind Doctor Jo that symmetry is a big part of beauty. They have put me on an antibiotic for it (could be a saliva gland); I am already on intravenous antibiotics anyway.

Thank you for your kindnesses, I am now at 11 nightdresses and so am nightied out; no I shall not be accepting the offer of having *lots of books* sent to me by a 'flibberty gibbet' in her 30s (you know who you are) as I am well into my bloodthirsty trilogy on the Vikings – at least in the days when I had time to read. The most bizarre offer was from my niece who offered to visit me from Wales. She is due to give birth in a few days – I asked if she'd be getting 1 ticket on the way up, and 2 on the way down and she replied that her partner would bring her in the truck. 'Decline' button pressed again.

Seriously, *everyone* wants to help but there's very

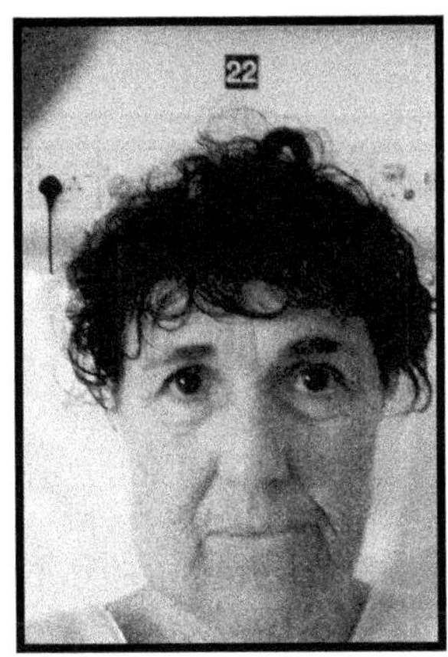

Asymmetric.

little you can practically do and from tomorrow I will need to wind down communication as 'ding dong' the fight begins, so don't expect individual replies. Coping with everyone's emotions is also hard (my parents have been very good), although it's been interesting hearing tough people say how much they love, and care for me!

School bookings are almost finished for the term so that will be a lot less work, although supplying an Egyptian string player for Oxford's Ashmolean Museum (they can't have the vibration of a drum you know); a Dancer I've never met to substitute me in Southend; and a team of 3 to Southampton, have been challenges I've enjoyed this week. After half-term is strangely quiet.

Who knows I may even get to read that newspaper!

'Do not go gentle into that good night . . . rage, rage against the dying of the light' wrote the Welsh poet Dylan Thomas – I hope to go into it for resurrection, one way or another,

Love,
Hazel

Friends 3

Dear All,

My last communication was sent bravely marching off to war singing, whilst being festooned by your flowers. This communication is not exactly from the trenches, but we have now entered the battlefield, talked to the wounded & been involved in minor skirmishes.

Short ending:

Symmetry now reigning in my face & lips restored to pink. Second full day of chemo: out of the 5 pages of side-effects – I feel a bit sick but hair still where it should be. Revived by 2 pints of someone's blood; if any of you fit Readers are *not* blood donors, *don't* feel guilty – just bloody well go and do it!

Longer ending (for those with nothing better to do):

Actually, some of your flowers have been somewhat wreath-like (although I know well meant) – 'We felt *rather sober* after reading up on your condition', and another, 'That is probably the worst news anyone can receive'. But with my dark Welsh sense of humour, these made me laugh – and I enjoyed them a lot more than some of the 'you'll be *fine*' ones. Both categories remind me that Job's friends ('Job's comforters') were actually a great help for the *first* 7 days as they sat in the dust with him – in silence.

Lots of you are confident because you say I am a strong personality – but I am reminded of when I had a wind-surfing lesson; I was an *excellent* pupil on dry land (teachers are), they even gave me *a bigger board*, only to be a complete physical flop once on the water!

Jayne my sister visited from Wales yesterday. She agrees this is the best hospital to be in (well they've been practising since the 12th century, so they must've got some things right by now). She also visited the Tower of London to see the 888,246 ceramic poppy cascade. An unexpected treat for her was being tested for matching bone marrow. Only 1 in 4 siblings is; one reason to have a big family. (Who came up with that saying I've always enjoyed that, 'Happiness is having a large and loving family – in another town'?)

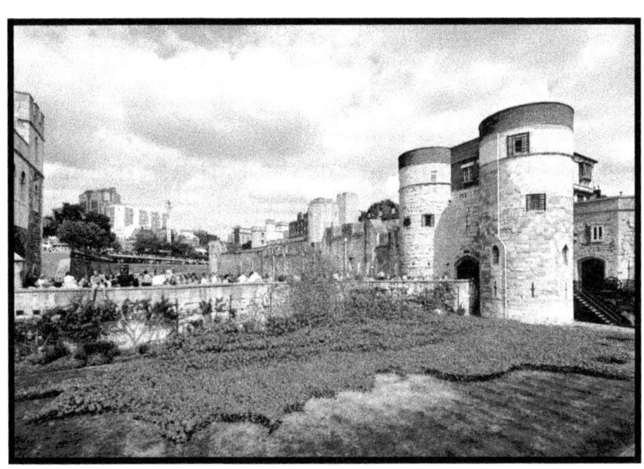

A poppy for every British & Colonial serviceman killed in WW2.

Our ward is still 'Closed' – despite swabs proving *no one* has a cold and the person, who *thought* they may be getting one, having gone home. This is because it was *a Nurse* who announced it 'Open'; whereupon *the Office* took exception & extended the closure to Sunday. No comment.

People are still allowed to enter but we can't leave. There's nowhere to go anyway except to the dayroom and meet a bunch of sick men. Oh yes there's a pile of books there too, probably left by 30-year-old 'flibberty gibbets'.

Quieter now, just 2 in the ward (well, no new admittance would want to get a hypothetical cold!). Who knows I may even get chance to clean out my handbag – a week ago I had a few biscuits in there, now I have crumble. My biggest fear is of it falling open on the floor in front of the very nice doctors, registrars (whatever they are for), nurses, etc.

Strictly Come Dancing tonight – definitely no visitors allowed!

Hazel

P.S. Still perfecting the art of the advice in the leaflet to 'lie flat and drink plenty of liquid'.

Friends 4

Hi Friends,

Sorry if not replied to any of you, *mostly* keeping up. Thanks for cards – a friend even rang from Australia last night but as I was watching Coronation Street, I didn't take the call, one has to have some standards you know (I *would* have, if I'd realised long distance though!)

Short ending:

Day 5 (of 10 of chemo). We are advancing into enemy territory. Not been hit yet but aware of the possibilities.

Long ending:

The battle plan is drastic but without any treatment, my war would have been 'over by Christmas' – so no alternative:

- To *kill* all the white blood cells in the blood for 10 days (you will remember the analogy of being rescued by the Americans – there is no discriminating SAS version as yet).
- Then there will be 3 down days, without resistance.
- Followed by 3 up days, when the body should recover.
- After a week or so off, this is all repeated another 2 or 3 times for shorter times.
- If no sign of cancer cells for 5 years this is called a 'cure'.

But as Helmuth von Moltke the Elder said, '*No plan*

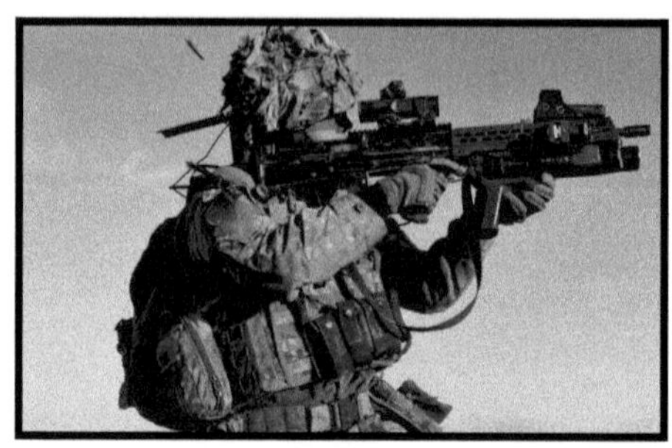

Homed in on target.

survives contact with the enemy' – and I don't want to be called to account for not following this ideal scenario, by disappearing down one of the many side routes e.g.:

- may get infection *'Do not pass Go. Do not collect £200'*.

- body may not start producing those cells and thus the South Somali woman in the bed opposite spent 2½ months in hospital on Round 1 (you see doctors are good at killing things, or chopping them off, but they cannot *create* the new cells. An interesting point). *'Miss lots of Go's'*.

- any other nasty may occur. *'Take a Chance card'*.

Present position:

Having extra tablet which makes me drowsy to avoid sickness – I reckon the payoff is worth it. Left arm swollen due to tube – had semi-permanent line put in today, unfortunately therefore had to be in *right* arm so will have to become ambidextrous in showering!

News from x-ray: my PICC line inserted from arm to chest has arrived at correct position (& from Me, the news that none of this has hurt!)

Hot off press from Consultant: my chromosomes are 'something or other' that is good.

Also of mention in this dispatch:

- Had visitors from church again today and I was able to take them up to 7th floor to chat, great view over London roofs!

- The ward is now officially 'Open' again & I have been to see the handful of books in the day room: they include these titles:

- *This Body of Death*.
- *Shroud for a Nightingale* (featuring a large picture of an injection held in a plastic gloved hand).
- *Oh Dear Sylvia* (about a woman dying in hospital).

When I did my Masters, I collected a list of the 10 funniest titles I could find on Africa: might do similar list of the most dire here.

Met one of the sick men from Essex. The ad '*No one should face cancer alone*' came on the telly: 'I neva used to fink anything of them ads', he commented.

Fink on Readers & do what really needs doing,

H

Friends 5

Dear All,

Hope those in education have enjoyed half-term; don't worry, those with children – they're back Monday!

The company here is good – 3 other women and we all get on. Last weekend we were only 2 – Terri an ex-Scottish Sword dance teacher & myself. We thoroughly enjoyed my friend's cake & 'Strictly Come Dancing'!

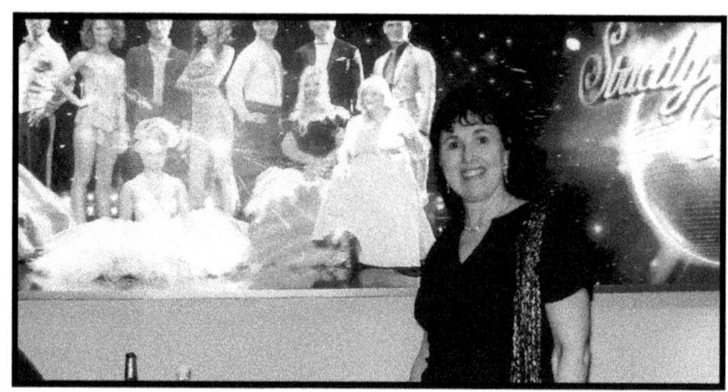

At the live Strictly show in 2010 – the night Ann Widdecombe went out!

Short ending:

It must be near end of this 'round' of chemo (leaving the timings to the professionals). I am, like a boxer however, not coming out *unscathed* (swollen arm & 2 blood clots in minor vein). The decision has been made to not treat them except with extra blood (& extra prayer chaps). They are out looking for a Vampire as we speak.

But the Commentator says I'm *doing well*.

Long ending:

Apparently, Prof Cavenagh is the 3rd best in UK – so one of the sick guys (the type who'd be interested in finding these things out) told me – actually he's *the head of infant car safety research* at Fords. That is the fellow patient – it's not the Prof's *sideline*. 'I always enjoy talking to you', he said (the Prof that is – try to keep up), as being Irish he enjoys my sense of humour. Mind you – he can do *putdowns* too; one of the nurses (the one who keeps sympathising & cooing over me like a dove) asked with a tremor in her voice if my swollen arm *hurt* to which he curtly answered, '*Of course it does*!' (this after I'd just finished telling him it didn't). I'm not sure he's the Number 1 fan of that approach.

Thanks for all the emails & texts. I loved this one from Metin a Turkish guy involved in the movie industry, worked on Lara Croft, etc: 'Hi my friend, I don't know what to say . . . but I know that You are very strong Lady. World traveller fighter Woman. You will beat that as well very soon. Our heart is with you all the time.'

Another wrote: 'I can't imagine a world without Hazel in it!' Bit of a dramatic statement but very sweet of her. Who knows it could be a better place! And on a *serious* note, lots of you have reason to know that, '*The graveyard is full of indispensable* people'.

Lastly, I have told another dear friend that I would mention her offer of bringing in 'Good Housekeeping' magazine. Comment superfluous.

I have not yet started losing hair, but in preparation I've chosen 4 designs which the wig lady will bring next week. She told me £50 for the quality I wanted, but said I don't have to pay when realised I was over 60 (just showing off, while I have the chance). It's quite a decision – should I go for something that would look good for dancing, if I should do that again? Have a complete change? (But there's nothing punky in the book.) Find the nearest match to what I have now? Or finally, go for short, which will best match my new hair? That's without the issue of colour – will I continue to dye my hair, or is this the time to reveal the truth, dear Friends? Answers on a £10 note (that pays for 7 days bedside telly).

Wondering how that musician I booked for the museum in Oxford will go down tonight at their Tutankhamen event. Wish I was there – still, Corrie on TV tonight.

Well can't wish you a Happy Halloween as not a fan, but as the origin is actually All Souls' Night, perhaps think about a quality you admired of someone who's 'gone before' – 'Sincere admiration leads to imitation'.

From,
Hazel (never spent a night in hospital until 2 weeks ago) King

Friends 6

Dear All,

I've appreciated the visits & phone calls of friends in Wales to my parents – who have both continued to be marvellous. We speak every day.

Short ending:

We are sitting low in the trenches hoping bullets fly overhead. My current course of chemo finished yesterday – I now have no relevant white blood cells as ammunition!

It's like the siege of Kobane (*for those who watch the news*) when its Kurds couldn't hold it, it's been invaded by their own Peshmerga and bombed from above by other forces. I will now be very vulnerable to infection until my own body creates new white cells. On subsequent rounds of chemo, the troops will be going house to house looking for snipers in various bones' marrow.

Caustic red chemo inadvertently inserted in arm, is now reaching surface, good. Blood clots still in place – they had their chance of escape with my thin blood. It's now been thickened with drip & so far not had any of the unpleasant mentioned side effects.

Long ending:

It's been great company being on this ward. Watched Strictly again on Saturday with Terri – this time in the Day

Room with bigger TV. I went in *earlier* & disenchanted the male patients of any notion that there'd be any other channel on at 6.30.

We planned to watch Strictly Results show last night together too – but I was on that platelet drip for which you have to lie flat, with an arm straight out (fortunately without having to 'drink plenty' simultaneously). Nurse forced it through & able to join her for dance-off.

2 of the women's husbands stay *most of the day* – their conversation gets very minutia-like. I am hoping to play crib with Terri & her husband later. She's been a good friend to me.

The nurses too are really good and very interactive. However, their *reactions* are not always encouraging – naturally some of this is because they are so much younger; for example, one of them commented that when you are my age, you can *teach* the dance but not *perform* (I kept quiet about having performed the week before). Yesterday when I was chatting with a Nigerian nurse about places we knew in Nigeria & America, etc, she ended with, 'And now you have your *memories*'. On this occasion I did speak up and say 'I've just been talking with this fellow patient & her husband about their trip to Abu Simbel in Egypt – *and I'm thinking of going myself*!'

Thanks to all of you who have told me what to eat for my good. No doubt some of the ideas will filter in. The food here is very good by the way (sounds like I should write 'Wish you were here' as my next line!) – milk shake & ice cream trolley most afternoons!

One funny thing – last Wednesday I was awoken from a deep sleep with the call 'Breakfast Club!' Butlins-like, the walking wounded were summoned to the Day Room, where we were treated to M&S fresh orange *with bits*, croissants, French bread, and coffee in a percolator!! All courtesy of the Mauritian Ward Manager who pays for it himself! May God bless him! I find myself child/Xmas-like waking up each morning & wondering – could it be *Wednesday*!

God bless you all with your busy Monday to Friday,

Hazel

Friends 8
(somehow there was no Friends 7)

Last night I got 'trench fever'. I wasn't shivering – I was *shuddering*, they call it the rigors (just googled the spelling of that & came up with 'rigor mortis'; well it wasn't that bad!)

The Ward Manager asked if I knew *what this meant*, I said 'YES, I may not be able to go to Breakfast Club!' Don't think the Mauritian gets my humour yet (not like the Irish Prof). Actually, it was a *genuine* concern, especially that the ward would be closed & the other 2 not able to attend. (Am I institutionalised?)

Today after more antibiotic drips I'm feeling fine; temperature down from 39.3 to normal. PTL

It was nevertheless a scary feeling – 1 in 20 die of infections you may recall from an earlier email.

Ah, the walking wounded are being summoned – 'Breakfast Club' . . .

Friends 9

Dear All,

A close friend asked how I 'really felt' apart from expressed in my literary efforts – well *this is* how I really feel. No pretence – if I were in pain you would see another side of me, but I am not. There is no fear – it's a win/win situation – to die is to be with my Creator who covered the *gone-off parts* of my totality with his blood freely given. To live is to delay, so as to be with my parents (in their late 80s) for their hour of need; and to work on that autobiography. Who knows, to travel more perhaps? I said to my many times travel companion in September, (as the saying goes) *Shall we 'see Rome and die'*? 3 weeks ago I thought I might have to leave out the Rome bit! But who knows?

Very short ending:

All quiet on the Western Front! Today I feel fine, normal even.

Short ending:

Blood cleared of *baddy* white cells (along with the *goodies*), & the marrow too ('We imagine' Prof said). But you wouldn't choose Kobane for a stroll – the whole process will be repeated more than once to be sure.

Terri opposite laconically queried whether my term 'trench fever' was a mixture of 'trench foot' and 'cabin fever'? (She could probably write this blog!) Anyway, it's threatened to come back twice, but I got the Paracetamol before shivering turned to shuddering. I've been left with no permanent tremor – unlike the many shell-shocked poor young men in WW1.

Battle scars: blood clots still there, but forgotten about them; arm where chemo got inside, angry red patch smaller & working to surface. By the time special cream arrives at pharmacy, the job of internal healing may be complete!

Longer ending:

So I am now at my lowest point in terms of vulnerability to infections. This at least has given me the excuse to ward off the nurse who coos over me!

Another nurse was coughing & sniffling 2 days ago, and I tried to get her reassigned or sent home. The answer was that she had had a lot of sick time and was in danger of going to the next stage in disciplinary procedures (maybe someone so sickly may be better off on a less vulnerable ward though?) When Pascal the Ward Manager returned in the pm, I spoke up again and she was sent home (surely being sent home should count differently to ringing in sick anyway). They are currently testing the source of my infection; I hope it's not related – I don't want to feel resentment.

But what you are all waiting to hear about, is of course 'Breakfast Club!' (Should this have any resonance in you, then *get a life*).

Pascal was late arriving with his goodies of fresh coffee, croissants etc (as he'd been here since midnight the night before although officially finishing at 3.30pm) & was amazed to see us tucking into bacon & boiled eggs. The Fireman, due to be discharged, had only got up early, gone to nearby Smithfield Market, then blagged his way into the Hospital hostel next door & cooked his fellow patients bacon & eggs. It was a glorious occasion – over-indulgence at which I suspect to be the cause of my one & only occasion of throwing up. I officially put it down to *drinking too much water for the fever* so as not to jeopardise the event!

There was another more intimate gathering on the 7th floor later as the 3 of us snuck up to watch the Bonfire Night fireworks, toasting them with pressed apple juice and fruit & nuts from that hamper I'd finally received that evening (8 days delay due to no ward number & for security the Postroom are not given our wards). We girls had fun, they hiding the goodies in their dressing gowns, while I pregnant-like, just for reassurance, held a sick bowl at the ready under my jacket.

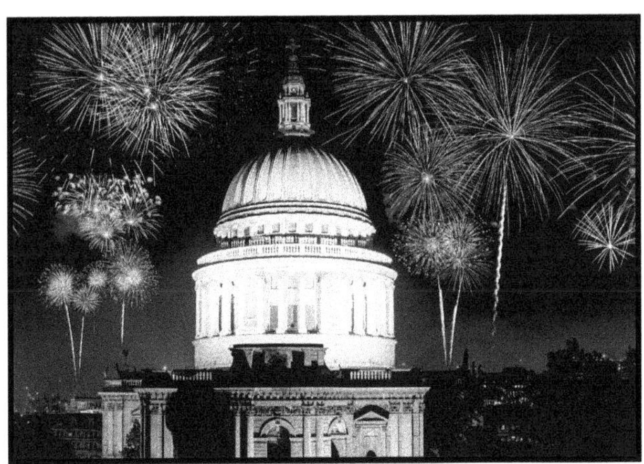

London fireworks.

We are 3 now as Mandy was removed to the Field Hospital (single room) couple of days ago due to infection.

It seems I misunderstood the timings; I may be here another 12 days. So those of you who were not lucky in receiving *tickets* to see me (& want to come) may be successful if reapplying.

I know not all of you like hospitals, so don't worry – likewise with hospital talk, just press delete as I have no unsubscribe button; hardly get round to putting more people *on* (yesterday 2 requests) & so slow with USB dongle as no Wi-Fi for patients.

If I make it through the battle tours, somewhere in the spring perhaps one of you young things could put these letters on-line under the title:

AML (*Acute Myeloid Leukaemia*) *Diary: do not read if have sense of humour bypass* (*Home Counties have been warned*).

But then if I come through, I could find out how to do it myself!

Enjoy the sunshine,

H

Friends 10

Dear Friends,

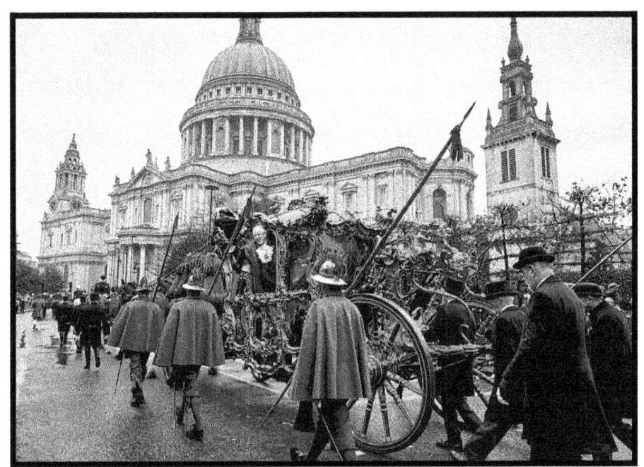

Lord Mayor's Show in all its glory!

I hope this message meets you all well rested. I had a great sleep last night, with dreams. You know *acceptance* of a situation comes at different levels. In my dream it had percolated through that there was a sick person standing there; *but it wasn't me*. In my 2nd dream I was on a bus in Hackney; a Jewish child in a party dress jumped off to join a celebration (*of which there are many – even 'Rejoicing for the Law'*). In her haste she left her coat & bag. I decided to get off at the next stop & walk back with them – then I realised that I *wasn't capable* of it.

Well I'll probably *end up* doing *all sorts* of things. Even today we had some excitement – some of the Lord Mayor's Show (for the benefit of overseas readers this is an enormous annual procession), was spotted from our ward window. It was only the stationary backside of 3 horses. I went up to the 7th floor but the view was away from St. Paul's. A man there told me it was visible outside the building – '*just cross a road*' – so Hazel left the building in Oct in T-shirt, leggings & slippers despite having heard that the temperature had really dropped since my admission. (We cannot experience it here in our space-age environment – there are no windows that open & air is filtered.) Discovering that it was down yet another road & corner, caution eventually conquered determination (most would call it *stupidity* for someone who presently has to avoid crowds).

Shorter ending:

We are all now looking for the first indication of my blood producing white cells (when I have those I won't be vulnerable) it has to be 0.5 of something or other before I can go home. At present zero. The doctors have done their preparations by killing the old & have improved conditions for the likelihood of the new – but as they say in the Strictly dance-offs, 'You have done your *best*, you can do *no more*'. They too stand and wait.

A couple of days ago, a friend of mine quoted the saying 'The horses are made ready for it, but victory belongs to the Lord' (reminds me of the groomed horses carrying red-coated Guardsmen that I saw today looking down at the side street waiting to join the procession).

I hope any *remaining* old cells in the blood will have as forceful a reaction as my great niece this week who, on Day 1 of sharing her house with the invader (her new sister) declared:

Nobody loves me!
Nobody wants me!
I'm leaving!

Now there's a girl who'll never suffer depression through not expressing herself!

Long ending:

Fevers: now gone. No infection could be identified as the cause of my *rigours* (not *rigors* at all). I suspect hysteria: possibly the doctors did too, as I notice I was never carted off to a side room like Amanda nor did the ward get 'closed' again.

Hand: effectively having suffered a 2nd degree burn is clearing up nicely.

Visitors: as there's *no time to say all this* before you've managed to break one of the rules (apart from no visit is possible if you have sniffles or 'the runs') . . . there is no kissing nor placing any item from the floor on my bed or table (surfaces apparently more deadly than people). Your own bags can go on the floor. With all this care, the drugs, staff, and medication, you can see why Leukaemia is probably simply a death sentence in any part of Africa (apart from S Africa).

Lastly do take care to not exit by the wrong lift. One visitor later emailed her experience on Halloween Night:

I had an adventure on the way out as I took a different set of lifts that took me down to a spooky area of the hospital . . . totally deserted and no way out!!! It was sort of fun!!! I had this image of me being trapped in empty floors and spending the All Souls Night going up and down the lift, looking for another human being!!!! Eventually, thanks to a man delivering goods, I was shown the appropriate lifts and I was saved!!!

I now have 32 cards to date & thanks to all I haven't got round to thanking – could I suggest that there's no need for any more (or if you must, put a Christmas card in with them to save a stamp!)

My next question for Prof Cavenagh, is whether he is sure *he's not doing a top rate job on the 'electrics', but the vehicle's a write-off*! I've touched on this before – the need of a super team of Consultants who look at the body as a whole. It concerns me that when a lymph gland swelled in August, & spectacularly in October, the cells may have travelled. I bounced this off a young doctor and am still contemplating my understanding of her explanation that in a cancer like Leukaemia, its own cells have turned rogue, rather than a cancer having arisen. Anyway, no harm those of you who are Prayer Warriors cutting off any troops that may have fled to another battlefield.

Life in the flat is going fine I am given to understand. One lodger sent a text to hurry back to do the *cleaning, washing & ironing*. Ha ha I replied, the other lodger told me *you* did the laundry. The reality turns out to be that he put the washing from the basket into the machine, and then came for further instructions. Put it back in the basket he was told by me!

Terri left 2 days ago; it was fun having her – may see her again on another of our rounds. Since then we've had 4 other patients pass through on their ways home. They all have their black suitcases on wheels and sit ready to exit, like on 'The Apprentice' show.

Another peaceful night – just Deborah & myself. Not being attached to a drip (had a 12hr one the other night with 2 bags simultaneously) makes it a lot easier to make the loo. Otherwise one has to unplug from the wall & push the drip stand (some of which behave like wonky supermarket trolleys) along with you. Should the bathroom door be lower than the drip stand, it requires the skill of entering as a pole vaulter. All a challenge for a middle-aged woman being pumped full of liquid! Some Readers are going 'Too much information', whilst others are sharing *deep sympathy* at this point.

By the way, if anyone has Friends 7 email can they send a copy back to me – I suspect it may not have existed. If you're reading this Saturday night, could you not find something more active to do? If on a Sunday, perhaps you're recovering from the activities of last evening!

As I write, the Lord Mayor's fireworks on the Thames are *blasting* away (but no rush up to the 7th floor – main windows face north!) Pray my levels go up W-H-O-O-S-H *just* like that!

Regards,
Hazel

Friends 11

Hi Guys,

Today for the first time I feel a bit down: 2 new people in the ward and lots of beeps of machines didn't contribute to good night's sleep; and the news was that the white blood level (of neutrophils) was still at zero, & Prof said it could take another 9 days to reappear! Don't feel like writing but with 30 on the list, people are starting to make their enquiries for news, and this is so much easier.

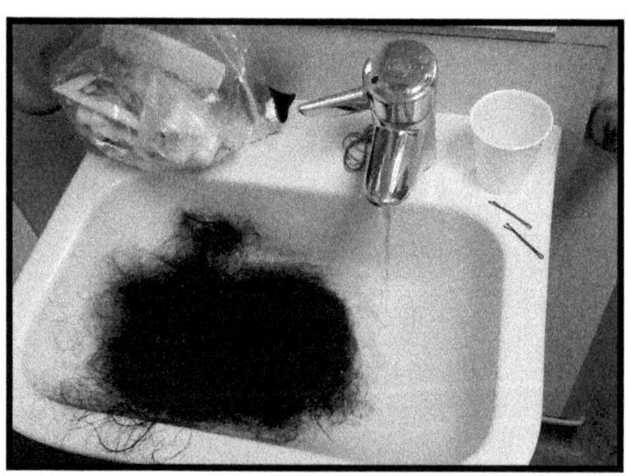

The collateral damage of Bad Hair Day!

Yesterday I was OK, despite it being Bad Hair Day to end all BHDs.

- I started the day with hair.
- 1hr later it largely all fell off & what was left I cut off (less now than my 1-week-old great niece's).
- An hour later wig lady arrived & I have full head of

hair again (actually too hot for in here, so wearing little caps – very 'Stamford Hill'; the Hasidic community.)

My lodger bizarrely suggested tattooing 'a rabbit' on my head. Why Phil? 'Well because from a distance it would look like a little *hare*!' The trials of a landlady!

Tomorrow my niece is coming & what with it being Breakfast Club and The Apprentice on TV, hopefully my spirits will pick up.

Short ending:

Even for someone so fascinated by themselves, I'm getting bored now of talking about me & my illness and feel like an over-indulged celebrity in a health spa, or wealthy wife in purdah, with all the attention from yourselves & the staff here – e.g. I'm monitored for blood pressure & temperature 4x a day – and have even put on weight.

Decided I will not be writing an email on subsequent visits – this round had some novelty value.

Longer ending:

I think I mentioned my 1st 2 visitors independently ended up in A&E that very week, now my 3rd visitor is in Barts himself. Reminiscent rather of the Howard Carter expedition. But don't let this put anyone off . . .

My diet is supposed to be restricted now I haven't any resistance to infection, but broke rules today to eat a crisp unpeeled pear & got caught by my special nurse! However, waking in the night, I really felt like a glass of milk from my fridge and a date & walnut bar. Remembering that nuts & dried fruit were not allowed under level 0.2, I at least did substitute it for a hygienic KitKat – kind of weird, isn't it!

We are only 24 beds in Ward 4a: two other bays like mine of 4 beds, and the rest side rooms. One man was transferred to Intensive Care. Amanda never came back but I wave to her through her door as I pass by: been passing by a lot as joined a male patient in his exercise route of 10 laps of the ward. After being in bed for 5 weeks he had not been able to stand; now the 10 laps gave him a foot blister! He's one of the 2 patients I saw when I arrived (it's so space-age you hardly see another patient) and *wished I hadn't* – he put me in mind of a Belsen survivor – but now he's become a nice guy I know and I'll miss him when he leaves tonight (badly timed, will miss Breakfast Club!)

Forgive lack of jokes, they are not flowing tonight.

Let's say something not about me to end – join me in thanking God the Lord Mayor's Show and the Armistice both went off without any bombings!

Hazel

Friends 12

Dear All,

Well I'm afraid no news is no news on those elusive levels, and when there is some you will all surely hear.

I am allergic to waiting (especially when I had the wrong understanding of timescale – it could be another week) – definitely more a person of action.

Today I have had major problems with laptop which I've been on for most of the day – the trouble with the email on a mobile is that you can't send mass email, nor a file. Seem to have fixed it with system restore but still not good.

The delay has resulted in lots of you emailing to see what's occurring – but I'm ok and have 2 different friends visiting tomorrow. But I'm going to try to relax for the weekend (and the weekend starts now), so kindly hold back on those emails and I may be able to read a magazine like normal patients. I know you're all concerned and value all your kind thoughts.

Regards,
Hazel

Friends 13

Good news . . . (to be sung to football tune '1 – nil'):

0.1
0.1
0.1
0.1
0.1
0.1
0.1
0.1

That's the news on the return of the neutrophils part of the blood that fights infection.

It's been 0 since finished chemo and this is the first sign of its return! I will be less vulnerable to infection as it increases.

When it reaches 0.5, I can go out of hospital for a week . . . before having to do it all again (don't worry, I've promised no emails then on).

Thanks for all your good wishes and prayers!

Regards,
Hazel

Friends 14

Getting ready to *'go over the top'* and come out! It has been tedious lying low hiding in the trenches waiting for ammunition (I hope you all saw 'Warhorse' on TV last night) and I know this has been reflected in the level of humour so many of you enjoyed. I loved this comment from one of my Readers though:

You may find, like Woody Allen, that some people prefer your "early, funny, stuff", but personally I feel privileged to have you share your thoughts and reflections.

Actually I suspect some never recognised the jokes when they came – after all my email has gone from friends in Australia to South Africa; and I recently learnt it was being forwarded to Cambodia. However, it is still probably the Home Counties crowd who would benefit from a special version with 'lol' added at appropriate points.

Anyway, my level of what fights infection is now 0.7 (which is a third of a person's normal level), so shortly *the whistle will blow*, and up the ladders we will go, to meet all those germs, virus, and disease in the world beyond Luke Ward at St Bartholomew's Hospital. (I don't mind telling you it's a little scary.)

This will naturally not be much in the way of a holiday, & unfortunately I may not get to Wales for long in my week off (if at all) as I have to come in as a day patient a couple of times for tests. I have been in email touch with my friend from the other bed who left 10 days ago. She has had to come back in for platelets & blood, so not much of a break if I'm like that (my account at this stage is still in the positive for the pints I've donated in the past I'm pleased to say).

So I'm expecting a rucksack of medications before going over – even learnt to *inject myself*, something I *never* thought I'd be able to face, but who else is going to do it – the lodgers & my mum? When there's no choice it's surprising what you can do.

My final email will just be a blast of a whistle, to let you know I'm dodging my way through 'No Man's Land'. I don't plan any further emails so will take the opportunity to thank each and every one of you for your kind thoughts, prayers, emails, phone calls, cards and visits. If I say I'm sorry to have taken up so much time in your busy lives, it might sound uncharacteristically humble, but that is how I feel.

Regards,
Hazel

Friends 15

Whoooooo!

Friends 15: extra dispatch

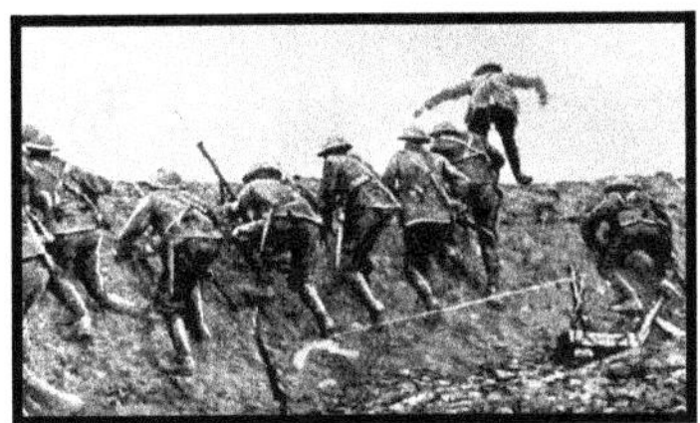

'Going over the top' WW1.

OK guys, so one Reader got it – that was the whistle in my last email calling me 'over the top'.

Accordingly I left the safety of the space-age capsule that is Barts' King George V building last night & came home.

My lodger fetched me and there was a bunch of flowers and bottle of wine waiting for the homecoming. So far, I'm fine.

All being well in tomorrow's tests I will be driving to Wales for a few days & back in hospital on 26th Nov.

That Reader - award yourself a campaign medal (for many of you have fought with me, & that one, to the end).

Those who didn't get it – no court-martialling at dawn for you, but you are condemned to solitary with only a copy of my hospital emails to read again.

H

Friends 16

This followed an email from my sister to the Barts email list:

Dear All,

Hazel has asked me to send a message to say that there has been a delay on her return to St. Barts as they currently do not have a bed for her. So, if you were intending to visit this weekend, please put on hold until further notice. She will be receiving some other treatment in the interim, so may not be contactable.

Many thanks for your continuing support,

Jayne
(*Hazel's sister*)

Hi Friends, etc,

Sorry you've had a long wait & lot of confusion – resulting from me in one hosp, & my luggage (with phone charger, computer, etc.) in another, so communication was tough – also someone going to the wrong hosp to visit me, & another enquiring at a hosp in Wales! They seek her here, they seek her there . . .

Where am I?

I'm up a gum tree backwards!

Got to Wales & had nice visit with my folks including seeing my new great niece. On return I had my bone marrow tested but the result, which will determine my next treatment, was not clear & I was due to repeat it Wed!

There were no beds so I was not admitted. Meanwhile I developed a high temperature due to little resistance to infection, so last Fri I was admitted to my local hospital, Homerton.

I'm now being treated with antibiotic drips; the bone marrow test being put to some point in the future. (If you remember, infection sees off 5% of Leukaemia would-be survivors.)

After 2 days on the ward with people coughing & shouting out, I'm thankfully in a side room so I don't get anything worse!

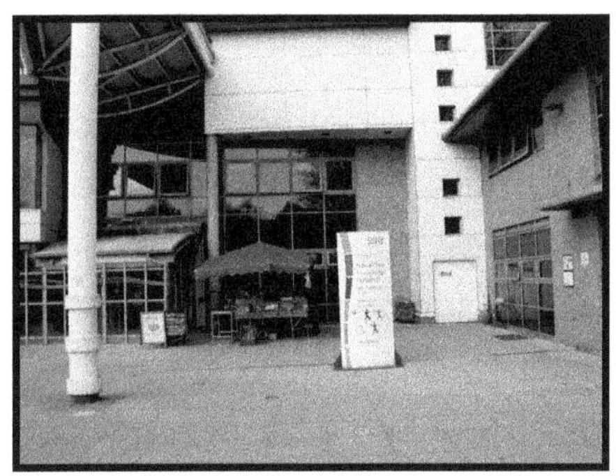

Back to Homerton – the forecourt where the A&E Dr came out to find me last Oct!

Readers, it's like this: when I returned from Wales I really didn't want to go down that known road of chemo again. Now I just wish my feet were on that despised path, instead of down this side lane stuck in the mud, or up a gum tree . . .

Hazel

Friends 17

Dear Friends,

Not much change since my last communication but I find if I don't communicate for a few days your 'where are you/how are you?' messages come through. I know you are concerned but it's a busy time of year with lots for you to get on with.

I could say *I feel well*, and *I look well*. I'm nice & warm in a quiet side room, own loo & TV – cups of tea and trays of food appearing, and looked after kindly with lots of various people coming through that door to see to this, that & the other. I now have my luggage back from Barts hosp fetched by my lodger, so I have my laptop, clothes & Christmas cards to write.

In other words, I feel like a bit of a fraud – as if I'm taking up a space someone *really ill* could have!

However, on the other hand the bit that is unseen says *I'm not a well woman*. I am still being treated for an infection thought to be the cause of the high temperature I had when I came in to my local hospital last Friday (it's possible to hallucinate at that 39°!) & which returned 2 days ago, after we thought it had gone (& on that account I could have been sent home).

The bit that needs to improve is the white blood cells called neutrophils. These fight infection & having improved since I left Barts, have now gone down and down despite me injecting in the stomach every day. They will eventually go up the further one is away from chemo, but then by the same token so are the chances of the Leukaemia cells hidden in the marrow (terrorists in training) coming out & taking over again.

I cannot be considered for further chemo until these problems are sorted.

It's a waiting game (one accepts one goes down a few snakes in Snakes & Ladders before eventually arriving) but this one is time sensitive - Snakes & Ladders with a timer!

This afternoon I missed going to a wedding a few streets away. With a tear in my eye, I told my Consultant I was to be the *only* guest, besides 2 daughters, at the wedding of a terminally ill friend (I *had thought* about going AWOL). He agreed to me going in a taxi but returning if anyone there had a cough or cold. I rang in advance and 1 daughter had a cold, the other a chest infection. I don't mind taking risks but unfortunately that was just beyond sense.

How do I feel? Philosophical as ever - my friend visiting from Belfast used the word 'serenity' (possibly a contrast with home), but still not something one would usually associate with Hazel King. My choice is still to come out of the present troubles and be judged fit enough to face chemo again, so we really need Jesus the healer!

Hazel

Friends 19
(18 doesn't seem to exist)

Dear Friends,

I hope you are not all wearing yourselves out at this busy period and be too tired to appreciate the joy of Christmas when it comes.

Many of you have been confused as to where I am and where I'm going to be on a particular day, e.g. a day they'd like to visit, or where I'll be even on Christmas Day.

The trouble is, since leaving my local hospital, *I haven't known myself* – thus the delay in my response. Today I'm being admitted to Barts Ward 4a to start chemo and will be here around a month.

As there are *still* Leukaemia cells in the bone marrow (they've drilled into my hip 3 times now, thank God for anaesthetic!) they will now try *another* combination of chemo drugs.

It's not what they hoped for (0%), but I understand the 6% could have been worse.

They will now induce the birth of the Leukaemia cells from the marrow to the blood to effectively target them. For those of you accessing the information better from the military angle – we are going back to Kobane where significant numbers of insurgents are apparently hiding. This time we are carrying different weapons and going to call them out to a fight in the open. May God help us!

Hazel

Friends 20

Dear Readers,

Just a quickie to say for those visiting or sending things, I'm actually in Ward 4b (not 4a now)

King George V Building
St Bartholomew's Hospital
London
EC1A 7BE

It's just along corridor from 4a so I can visit Terri, the Scottish Sword dance teacher, who I was with before. Who knows perhaps we'll watch Strictly together on the big day room TV tonight! Out of the ones I was with before, 3 are doing well & 1 has died (Iris the East Ender).

I am here in 4b because I am having this different chemo – I am about to start when a drip stand is available (the ward is new & some teething problems!) I still feel a bit of a failure not having licked all the Leukaemia on the standard chemo but after a night's sleep I am more resigned to it.

This one is stronger and will involve a week of first calling the Leukaemia cells out of the marrow – whether we shall be simply calling out 'cowardy custard', or throwing in Molotov cocktails, I'm not quite sure.

Here we go!

Hazel

P.S. While at home I managed, away from the crowds, to greet 2 brides in 2 days!

P.P.S. I will think of you all in the Big Freeze as temperatures plummet, while I stay at constant here.

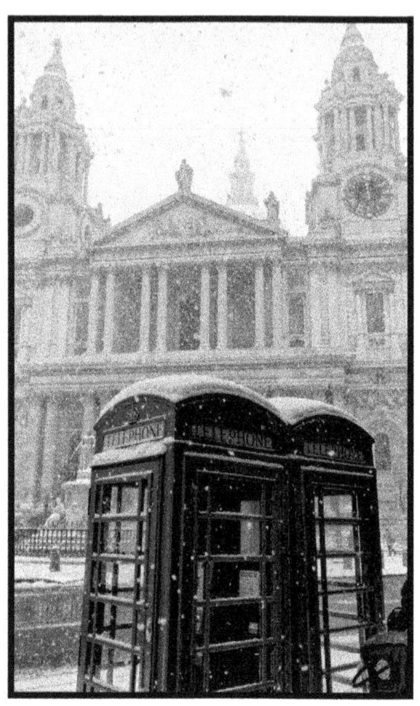

St Paul's when it snows.

Friends 21

Dear Friends,

I know some friends have been asking for more current information – possibly others will think, 'Not very seasonal these tales of illness!'

Well, for those who want to know, this is the 3rd day since they finished giving me chemo (it passed so quickly I didn't know it was over till the next day), however there will be a longer recovery time to this stronger chemo, so that is why I will be in until sometime in January. It is still coursing in my veins making me feel *pretty lousy* – I hope the Leukaemia cells feel worse!

I achieve very little in a day as opposed to my female friends who report frantically sorting this, that & the other for the deadline & going to events they are too tired to properly appreciate – while I read a slushy magazine just because I never do, chat to a young Bengali patient, try to fix people's TVs, etc.

Unless there's a visitor, or a programme I really want to see, I often *sleep* as when I'm asleep I don't feel the sickness. I have had a visitor a day on average (3 different people yesterday but none today, hence time for email) and this will continue until Christmas Eve when my friend will visit from Finland (like Father Christmas from the North, or the Wise Men from the East). In the understandably quiet period after that, who knows I may get time to write some of my autobiography – or I may join you all slobbing out with the telly!

I have a lovely position now by the window – see photo of view. (The other is a selfie of me having walked up to the Bara peat bogs in the summer). I enjoy the sight of the variety of building styles. However, my position near the window is under dual threat: the accelerating runs threaten to see me isolated in a side room, & also the whole ward may move to another building!

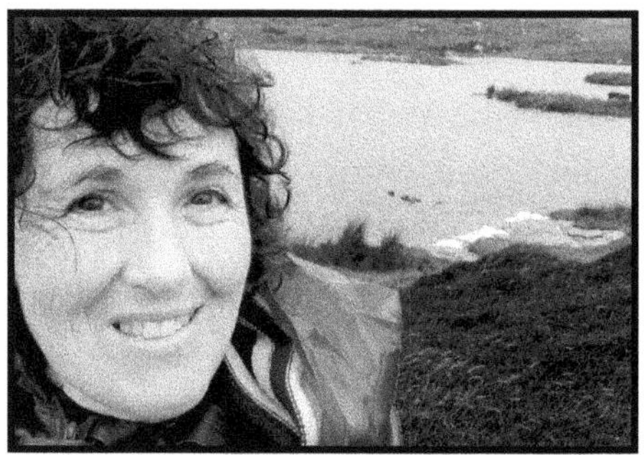

On the Scottish island of Bara
4 months ago looking good
but feeling lousy & not knowing why.

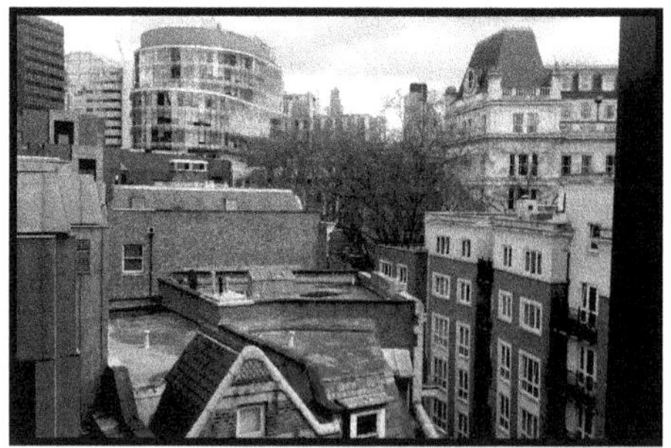

Current view.

Terri, my friend is doing *well*, she managed to stay on the other chemo (I missed the pass mark for residual % of cancer cells by I believe, 1 or 2%). She was 1 treatment ahead of me anyway, so having finished her 3rd course she is waiting to leave & hoping to be pronounced in remission. Meanwhile *my* goal is to stay awake tonight, not only for Strictly, but also for the later Results show!!!

We have a new Consultant now – a young woman on the job for the first time and she is brutal. I orchestrated at Breakfast Club for the Ward Manager to hear mine & the 3 other patients' stories, and he will speak with her. She has put down hopes & been certain of disasters – I have since challenged her yesterday when she said I *would* get an infection next. I said I hadn't had one *so far* [no temperature episode has come with proof of infection] & it was only the case that I *might* have one. Not everyone can fight like me – people here are vulnerable to being crushed in spirit particularly when they are here over Christmas.

I have never bluntly asked *my chances* – it was enough that Prof Cavenagh held out the *possibility* of cure – but on initially meeting me I could see that this woman was going to tell me however I might try to fend the information off. Anyway, it's not all bad, and there are some of you who will be wondering, so here it is: I have moved from *medium* to *high* risk (due to response to 1st chemo), but there's *more chance of me making it than not*, and lastly, that *remission is possible* on this chemo regime also.

Let's turn those words into *festive positives*: As mortals we are all at *high risk*, but we can *make it* to immortality through the *remission* on offer to all.

Yes, cancer is unforgiving – but that is *so unlike* the one who came to join us:

Jesus – God's selfie! ('He is the image of the unseen God': Col.1v15)

Hazel

Friends 22

Dear All,

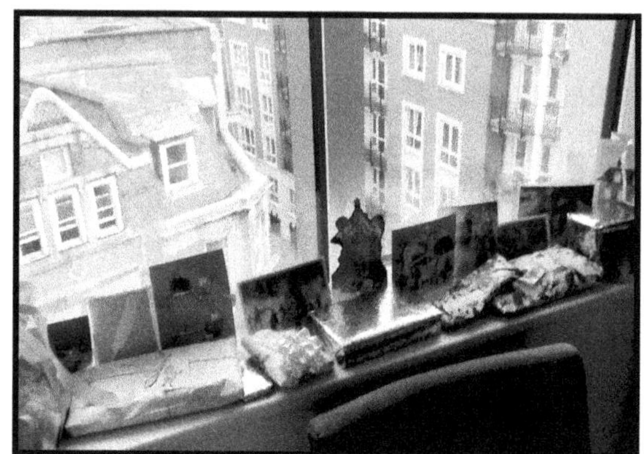

Christmas gifts on my window ledge.

Hope everyone had the Christmas they hoped for & are still relaxing in the rest of the 12 days!

Since my first Christmas gift of a pint of blood (giver anonymous), I've continued to receive & now must definitely be in donor debt after consideration of what I had paid in. I had lots of presents to open until I became tired & took a break, then found myself unwrapping presents at 11.30 at night to get it accomplished! By the way could you confirm on unnamed parcels – who actually gave me the *lavender cream, Serenity book, Lily O' Brien's chocs & the green poncho*.

This tiredness has continued & today I have been moved to a side ward because an infection has been discovered which might account for it. It is in the line that was inserted from my arm to near my heart which is very useful for avoiding injections. It is treated by the antibiotic I'm already on for temperature peaking & they don't seem unduly worried. It is irksome that the *assertion* of the new Consultant, that I *would* have an infection, has come to pass.

On the positive side, the side-effects of chemo seem to be passing – particularly the stomach problem & I'm eating more although not proper meals.

On the positive side of being in a room alone is not hearing the scrakey voice of the 90-year-old in the ward saying the same things all the time (she wasn't a bad woman at all) & the dreadful stench of the immobile woman alongside me, just 5yrs my senior, when she was changed. Without windows that open, the smell could last 2hrs.

On the down side is the fact that this room, which I suspect I am the first resident of, has not been fitted with a fridge yet; the TV connection is not working as it's the 1st room of what will be another ward & someone somewhere hasn't pressed a button (good job Strictly Final was last Sat as I couldn't even go to Day Room to watch as infectious) – and lastly, I have ensuite one of those trumpeting toilets, where an air block can cause the pipes to sound off for quite a few minutes after flushing!

Sorry can't think of any jokes,

Hazel

Friends 23

Dear Friends, etc.,

Happy New Year to you all! I hope this time next year finds you in a better place body, mind, or spirit.

Last night I was pleased I waited up for midnight as the Staff brought around Shloer 'wine', cakes & nibbles & were quite jolly. The noise of the fireworks would have woken me anyway, even with double glazing & being a bit down the Thames, it was like the Blitz! This area, around St. Paul's, was razed to the ground by fire in the war & it was like being transported back to then. If I'd found my gas mask, I'd have gone to the shelter.

My friend Terri, the ex-Scottish Sword dance teacher popped in to say she was going home that very evening.

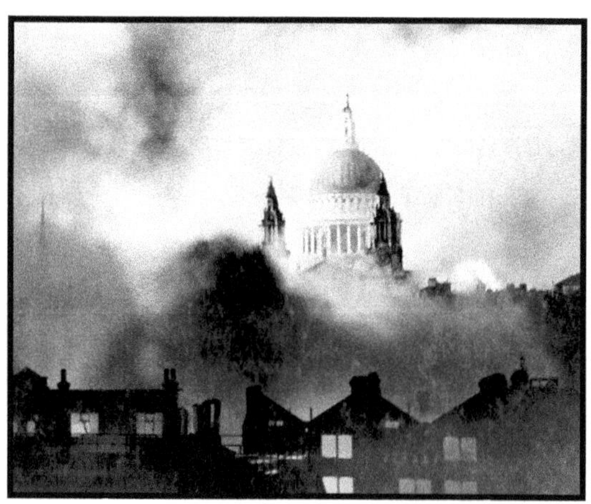

St. Paul's in the Blitz.

She's finished her treatment. I'm really pleased for her, as she wanted all the bad things to be in 2014.

On the positive side for myself, I have moved so far from the chemo that most side-effects are gone. I can eat a meal again (in the interim I had tried coaxing myself with a choice from the halal, kosher, West Indian & pureed menu – all to no effect!)

However, I am still in the side ward being treated for both the positive & negative version of a bug commonly found on the body: problem being it is in my arm line. The first antibiotic it was *resistant* to; so I am now on a very strong one. Should this not work, they will remove it – the line, not the arm. After so much antibiotic, someone will only need to whisper the word 'Superbug', and I'll keel over! *I think it best to put visitors off until the problem is sorted*.

My father is also in hospital but doing pretty well. Poor Jayne, how I wish we could have shared the caring of Mam & Dad this Christmas & at this time!

So this is the upshot: if I can get some neutrophil white blood cells returning, and also recover from the infection – I can come out and do lots of good & useful things, like file my tax return. Such aspirations!

As it is at present, I am just in bed (well I've made myself sit in a chair to write this as they've started checking my legs for blood clots now). Those of you who know me *well* will know that normally, as soon as I sit down at home, I jump up to do something or other I've thought of – you will find it strange *now* that between the decision to do something, & actually doing it, is a time lag of about 10 min! My biggest achievement of yesterday was changing my nail varnish to greet the new year. This morning I lifted 3 mop buckets of water to unblock the toilet & was exhausted. The ensuing 5 min of trumpeting in the pipes on flushing (that Terri & I thought was due to people drilling on the roof) is so bad, it means I don't like to disturb other rooms by flushing so often. Oops, overdid it this time!

Thank you to everyone who has given me a book, I am enjoying the J. John one on the Christmas story & I think it may be time now to finish my one on the Vikings in the continued absence of TV which has bothered me not a jot in the past week since I have slept through a lot of it (by the way, giver still not tracked for 1 item: lavender candle).

J. John comments on John the Baptist's parents' long-term childlessness may be of interest to any of you who has been thinking about 'the problem of suffering' lately: it's rather blunt but turns the question on its head:

'Throughout history, people have assumed that if you are good, God will be so pleased with you that only good things happen to you. Of course, it doesn't work like that. We all deserve nothing, and it is only because of God's grace that we get anything good at all. What is really surprising is not why bad things happen to good people, but why good things happen to any of us at all.'

Greetings to all!

Hazel

Friends 24

Friends, etc.,

Interestingly the quotation I used seems to have set off a little flurry of a discussion, contributions to which have been very varied. Let's see it again:

'Throughout history, people have assumed that if you are good, God will be so pleased with you that only good things happen to you. Of course, it doesn't work like that. We all deserve nothing, and it is only because of God's grace that we get anything good at all. What is really surprising is not why bad things happen to good people, but why good things happen to any of us at all.'

(Now to my mind it is *The Bad News*, without which *The Good News* of God's personal & costly intervention in history, makes no sense.)

OK so without mention of who said what, here are 3 very different responses from people of 3 different faiths:

- I didn't realize that Christianity was this negative!
- To me it reveals that although God is so very, very big, and we so very, very small nevertheless, we are so preciously loved by Him, greatly enjoyed by Him, and crowned with glory and honour.
- I am thinking of people who are beating themselves up because they feel that they brought the disease of cancer on themselves.They are non-smokers and

non-drinkers. Perhaps I should show them the quote re John the Baptist's parents.

That last quotation is with reference to the news breaking around the world today that 2 out of 3 cancers are due not to lifestyle, nor genes, but to '*bad luck*' (now isn't that just what my doctor told me weeks back!) Doesn't sound very scientific but perhaps relates again to that 'ability to dwell in uncertainty without the restless desire to know'.

Anyway I expect there are some *who still want to know* how I'm getting on!

There is some good news, the latest blood tests do not show signs of either infection!!!! This will have to be *confirmed* over time.

The bad news is that I *feel* worse, despite having a pint of someone's blood every day (mine can't be up to much!) This is due to the return of nausea after our cavalier experiment at dropping all 4 types of sickness tablets at the same time (plus I suspect I have a cold). Temperature still all over the place – fixing my shoes sent it over the 38º threshold.

The new Consultant now trying to cheer me up by saying it's the *hospital treatment* that has caused all these problems by aggressively trying to kill all the cells in every bone marrow. It's not my fault (same theme, not my fault, not God's . . . now we discover it's the hospital's!)

She is now much more human, however her cheery companion told me it could be 2 weeks before I see any return of neutrophils, along with discussions of coming out!

Dad's still kept in hospital; Mum can't visit due to a cold, so Jayne doing everything.

Some get all the practical work it seems, while others have time to lie here and philosophise,

Hazel

Friends 25

GOOD NEWS!

My count has kicked in – my own white blood cells that fight infection have started reappearing – 0.2 yesterday & 0.7 today; a normal person has between 2 & 7, so I'm at a tenth!

What with the good news about the infections going I *should* be feeling great – I *don't*, as I'm still on the heavy antibiotic & have *slept* all day. Coming off antibiotic soon. Have a number of visitors coming tomorrow, hope I don't drop off!

Think we'll round off the discussion basically of 'Why has Hazel got cancer?' The bigger issue being 'don't we deserve *good* things?'

This question is wrestled with by Job (possibly the oldest book in the Bible), as by my 4-year-old niece today when she looked back over her letter to Father Christmas and asked her mother why a couple of items were missing. So here's a friend's contribution:

Surely we can expect that a supposedly good God who has created us out of love owes us something? (*I don't think much of parents who create children and then don't do anything to make their life good – even if that, of course, might include setting them challenges and letting them misuse their freedom, etc.*) *To say that we deserve nothing may be technically correct, but it raises big questions about what kind of God has created us*!

The glory of God is human beings fully alive, not down-trodden ones who deserve nothing – we deserve everything! (*Yes, we are worth it*!)

God does owe us whatever – we did not ask to be created! (*playing the stroppy teenager*).

My own idea is that, *first of all*, if we – who act so rebelliously right in the face of an intense light that is God – if *we*, ask to be treated 'as we deserve', we should not be surprised if we are squashed by a big foot!

However, *secondly*, the amazing love of God treats us better than we deserve and many good things come our way.

Amongst mine I count the fact that:

- I spent 62 years without staying in hospital.
- During my treatment I have experienced no pain near toothache.
- No debilitation as bad as the *real* flu.
- I have received so many expressions of love of friends & family.

But, what about all our 'good deeds'? Well they exist, but like with the good blood cells, they *cannot balance out* even a few cells with Leukaemia, the latter will run the show.

Tonight is the last of the 12 nights of Christmas, so I will add that the *best* gift God gives is the offer of restored relationship with him, & each other. Please don't think I always *feel* that – & like every open-minded atheist, agnostic & those of other faiths, I have doubts from time to time. Perhaps that's healthy in a relationship,

Hazel

Friends 26

Dear All,

MORE GOOD NEWS: my liver, kidneys, etc. which could have been damaged by this strong chemo (temporarily or otherwise) have shown up as *fine* on the scan they take.

Ok now here's the *apology*: let out of hosp unexpectedly Wednesday & now it's Sunday and I've not let people know I'm home (this has resulted in 3 people going to the hosp to see me when I'm not there – I had known 2 were coming & texted to tell them: I didn't know their mobile was in the menders!)

So why the silence? – I was released due to *numbers* being good, but the person they related to *felt like* a dish rag & subsequently slept most of the time. Friday eve I revived – my lodger helped me get one of my favourite meals from Finsbury Park & he put on a Netflix 2012 comedy with Arabic music (I can't recommend it, it was too rude in places – 'What, *Hazel* recommended this!') & I heard myself belly laugh, for the first time in months.

Yesterday I checked myself in as a day patient at the hospital. When you are an inpatient, they check vital signs every few hours – then suddenly they say, '*OK you can go home for 5 days*'. It's just too long. I did need 2 pints of blood.

So here we are today Sun now, having woken up in the afternoon rather than the morning. Friend coming soon

& we are going to clean the flat – lodger surprised 'Why?' Actually, they've been very good, one doing my washing up one day, & the other the next! (I'm thinking of running training courses for wives).

Apologies over, where are we at? 2 courses of chemo down now, next week marrow from a bone will be extracted & the successfulness of the strong chemo will be known. Based on this will come the decision as to the next round.

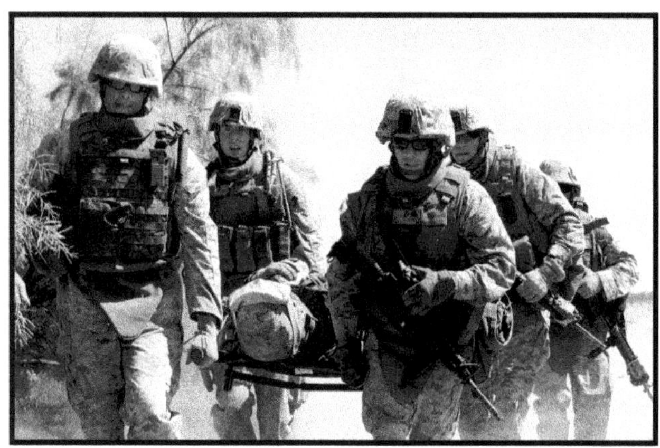

Rescue by the Americans.

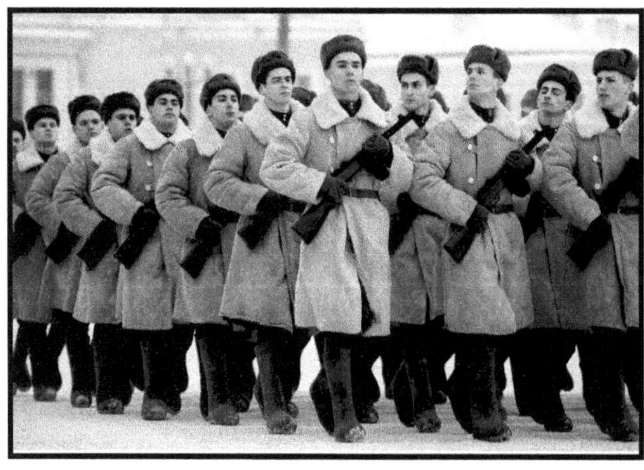

Rescue by the Russians.

I hope the Leukaemia cells felt as bad as me & actually died off. Whereas the 1st chemo was like being rescued by the Americans (all white blood cells killed off) this was more like rescue by the Russians (all white blood cells *plus* some of the red killed off).

Sometimes I think 'the lady does protest too much'. This morning I had an email with the line: '*Actually Hazel, I don't think I really have any idea of what you have been going through and how hard it is for you.*' Well it's not *painful* let me stress again, gruelling yes, gruelling but no pain. Every part is affected from the departure of my hair & eyes needing hydrating during chemo, down to toenails which now have chemo lines on them but are, on the positive side, *strong* now! Similarly, my anarchic eyebrows have been replaced by ladylike ones!

The situation this week for those who want to know: I am basically 'at home', unless whipped in; & in hospital as a day patient on Monday & Wednesday. Not a lot of time for fitting visitors in but don't let that put you off if you would like to come to the house (usual conditions apply, I'm up to the level of a wimp now – 2.0! PTL, but still no coughs & colds or physical contact).

Love to all,

Hazel

Friends 27

Dear Friends, etc.,

I am now in remission. No cancer was found in the bone marrow extract.

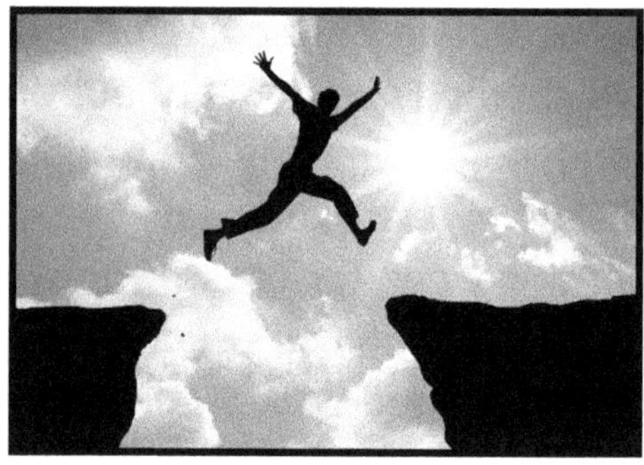

This is of course excellent news, only dampened by the fact I have to return to hospital on Tuesday to do the strong chemo all over again!

I will now go to Wales for a few days to see my parents who are now having carers as my sister has to go back to work.

Thanks for all your thoughts, wishes & prayers,

Hazel

Friends 28

Hazel would like her friends to know that she went back into St. Barts Hospital last night for her 3rd course of chemo. She will be in Ward 4a again. Any further information, e.g. full address, directions to St. Barts, and visiting times can be found on their website.

Hazel will probably be there about 3 weeks, depending on whether she gets an infection again during treatment. As always, to reduce risk to patients, please do not visit if you have a cold/cough/sickness, etc.

Regards,
Jayne

Friends 29

Dear Friends, etc.,

Greetings from Barts Hospital! (As my lodger's grand-daughter who visited asked, 'Where's *The Simpsons'* hospital then?')

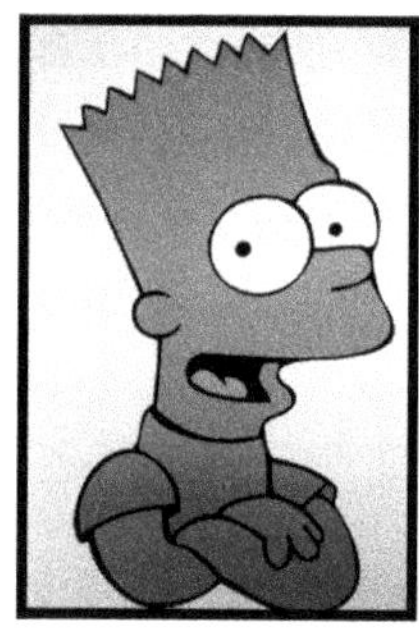

So we've *had* Round 3 of chemo and now it's going to take about 2 weeks to recover from the treatment. It's bizarre booking into hospital, apparently very healthy (having effortlessly been on 1hr country walk recently) knowing you have arrived to be reduced again to having to clean up the unplanned gross from every orifice (as from a giant baby) whilst feeling yuk & with temperatures up to 104.

I am protected from the cold blasts that those of you in UK are experiencing but feel cold & shivery enough when I get those fevers. But again, no pain; thank God.

Friends have come most days (one 3 days running!) and this would be a good opportunity for those who haven't visited but would like to. (This week would also be an excellent opportunity for the taxman to receive my tax file too of course!)

Thank you to all who sent me texts & cards, etc. for my 63rd birthday yesterday! Two friends visited, both with cakes.

At present, due to getting an infection immediately on arrival (one is supposed to get them after being brought down to zero resistance to infection), I am in a lovely private room within sight of a grassed rooftop which really lifts the spirits. Naturally I may soon be sent back to the ward, which was pretty miserable as none of the other 3 women spoke English, and one had constant visitors even overnight! But we just have to be glad for good things while we have them.

Best wishes to all,
Hazel

Friends 30

Dear All,

Thank you all so much for your support during the last 3½ months. I am now poised to return to normal life, whatever that was. Chemo is over: I do not have Leukaemia now.

Coincidentally, I heard this week that the town of Kobane (the siege of which I used as an image last Oct and some Readers latched onto) is now *totally secure*. Troops will no doubt be withdrawn now, just as I myself will leave hospital, but not until secure levels are reached (neutrophils above 0.5 in my case; at present zero).

This is all cause for rejoicing, but with the knowledge that we live in an evolving world – Kobane could be invaded again in the future; and I have *a very high chance* of developing Leukaemia again at some point.

Later I may have bone marrow ('stem cell') treatment which *may* increase *to even*, my chance of not having Leukaemia again. The treatment itself however also carries a 10% chance of death, so it's not something to be sneezed at. At present no donor has been found anyway.

Thank you to all who have visited, sent cards, texted, and emailed. Thank you also to those who have prayed or sought to pray for me. The hospital has been excellent – there have been 1 or 2 mistakes (the chemo burn on my arm is still purple) but they have been innocently made.

I've been very impressed with the approachability & humanity of the doctors & nurses.

I hope my life post this trauma will be worth your & their efforts.

Regards,
Hazel

Friends 31

Dear All,

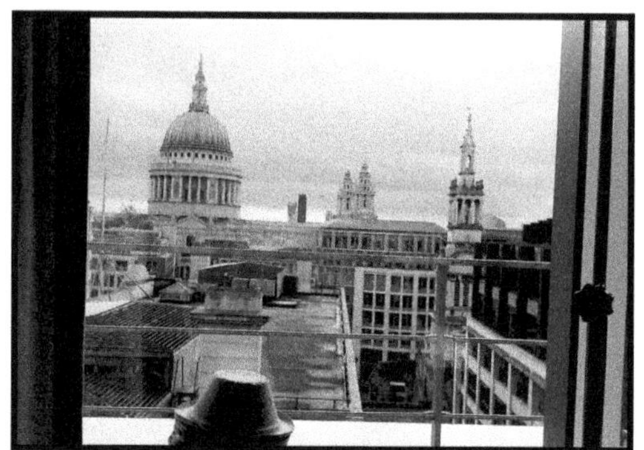

The dome of St Paul's Cathedral & the sick bowl domes.

This is the view I have from my outpatients' couch!

I have been out of hospital for 3 weeks now. Apart from a couple of infections and temperatures, I have been feeling very weak. However, a few days ago, I attended my only social function since October – 1hr of my friend's husband's wake!

Last week I couldn't walk the 5 steps from the sofa to my kitchen without huffing & puffing, which was pretty scary, but 3 pints of blood one day solved that.

All this had made me seriously question whether the Leukaemia had come back: I actually *felt* the same as before I was admitted from A&E last October which spooked me.

But to my delight today, the Consultant informs me

that I do not have cancer in my bone marrow extract. I don't have *much else* in there either – she called it an 'Empty Quarter' which might account for my lack of energy. (You may recall I likened the strong chemo I had to being rescued by the *Russians*: everybody is likely to get shot hostage included).

The fellow patients I've met today all feel tired too – in time to come, when advances are made, people will look back on this treatment as ridiculous.

So now we're going full steam ahead (a slightly optimistic image) for the stem cell treatment probably in April. My immune system will be taken down and someone else's uploaded. Naturally this is not without its dangers – but without it I only have 15% chance of the Leukaemia *not* returning within 5 years (& most likely in the 1st or 2nd year).

Amazingly there are 2 donors available & they are at present being tested for 'best match'. They are unlikely to share my blood group which is rare, so I may even find I change to theirs! My childhood injections will have to be redone – & I will lose the resistance I built up to elephantiasis in the tropics – but these are the least of my concerns.

I actually expect to be in Wales for Easter having been unable to make Mothers' Day, Dad's birthday, etc.

Resurrection.
Hazel

Friends 32

Dear All,

One knows it's time to write another general email when so many people start asking what's going on! What one has to appreciate however, is that I may not be saying what's going on simply because I don't know myself.

However, some news today.

The BIG STORY is of course . . . about the stem cell transplant.

There was a 2nd donor identified who amazingly is a 10/10 match to myself (this should aid by reducing the possibility of rejection). They came into the picture later than the 1st possible donor, so the earliest the operation process could begin, i.e. in 2 days' time, looked unlikely. I was imagining therefore *next* week (I've never even unpacked my suitcase) – but today the Anthony Nolan Trust said the donor wanted the end of *May*, meaning I wouldn't go into hospital until around 21st May to have my immune system taken down by chemo (I wonder if the guy is a teacher since he has requested half-term for his part in the matter?)

As well as protracting the period when one hopes Leukaemia does not return, it also means I will now definitely not make the family holiday on 12th June, as I will be in for a month at least. I broke the news today & we have to be philosophical about it & just put health first.

If all this goes ahead, interestingly I will likely be

changing blood group from a *universal recipient* (my rare group of AB negative) to this person's *universal donor* group of O positive.

Although the transfer of cells will only take about 1hr, the time in hospital is at least another 3 weeks. I *will* in these weeks be quite sick and *will* have infections (some of which are necessary to show the 2 immune systems fighting – hopefully not to the death!) It may be appropriate to have a reduced number of visitors. Not everyone will be able to hack it, and if I'm throwing up, I may myself be preoccupied. Also I will remain vulnerable to infection for 2 years, including to illnesses which my previous childhood injections once covered me for. After some months they can be repeated.

However, there is also a SUBPLOT . . .

Whereas one should be as fit as possible to endure the transplant, I have had 2 problems:

I've had difficulty walking due to tingling in my legs (& arms). Cause unknown – could be the chemo. At times I have looked like I am drunk in the street. But since yesterday there is a marked improvement in this & I can walk downstairs without grabbing the wall. I've even tried some running in my daily walk around the fields (well more like lolloping really) & not fallen over. Also a friend gave me a CD with a new version of the 'Rasputin' song & that has inspired me to want to dance! Dance isn't too difficult because when you wobble on one foot you just fall onto the other & act like it's deliberate!

The 2nd problem is still under investigation. Just before Easter I was told that the line from my arm to near my heart had slipped down & needed to be pulled back; so long as *nothing* was put into it, I could have it done on my next appointment. When I went to the hospital it was discovered to be a lot worse than they thought and the line was actually *in* my heart. Also, it had been in my left ventricle since *November* – no one had noticed on the x-ray and the doctor actually apologised. (When I saw the x-ray I didn't blame them, it looked very indistinct to me.) So, all the chemo, antibiotics, blood, fluid etc have gone straight into my heart for the *whole* of my treatment.

Well I'm *still here* to tell the tale, but now being investigated for arrhythmia of the heart since I have a buzzing particularly when I move. This could be something or it could be nothing. I had a 24hr monitor attached last week but the results may not be known for a while.

So that's the situation – bet you're sorry you asked now!

Meanwhile back to the hospital tomorrow for my hip to be drilled into for 5th time to see if still all clear. All 3 doctors I've had, agreed it's young men who feel the pain – the last doctor commenting that any time you see a young man enter looking like he'd look for a fight in a pub, you know you'll have trouble. Fortunately, being a *middle-aged* woman (I'm told *70* is now '*old*') I have no problem at all.

Greetings to all from Hazel!

Friends 33

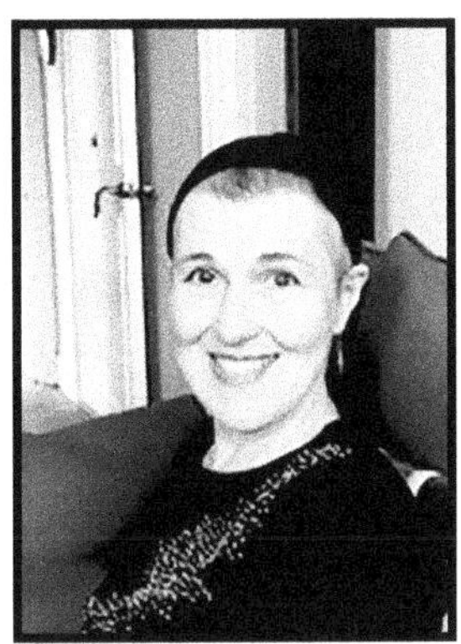

Stronger due to delay.

MAIN NEWS: the donor has been 'cleared' after his last tests (for HIV & STD) proved negative, so we go ahead. I will go into hospital on Thursday (21st May) for 5 days of chemo to remove my resistance not only to infection but also to foreign bodies; then after a 'Rest Day' the donor's stem cells will be introduced on 27th May. It works in just under 50% of the cases.

The 10% death rate is I believe spread over the following 2 years during which rejection can occur. Living or dying – *'a win-win situation'* as someone in church described it. Agreed. It is also true that I should like to live right now.

I will be in hospital at least a month. Anyone visiting should text first to find out if it's appropriate. Obviously, visitors with coughs, colds, etc. will not be able to visit – but also the patients I've seen having transplants have been *pretty sick* (literally that is) and also isolated with infections once the transplant occurs (24th May is scheduled to be medically a bad day as well).

Meanwhile I'm in very good health and back to my usual self. When people no longer stand up for you on the tube you know you *look good* too! A dear friend commented, 'It must be *harder* going into hospital when you feel so well!' How true! So I would appreciate not being contacted to 'see how I am' right now, as I feel *fine* and want to just enjoy being fit. (Also I'd like time to spend this week 'putting my house in order' with things in the flat and paperwork.)

I don't know if anyone watched 'The Big C' on TV, about a young woman who died of breast cancer. As she was writing a blog, I wondered if there were any common experiences. One thing I was interested in was her comment: '*Everyone wants to talk about illness and people say they're thinking about me all the time. It's very kind of them – but it's suffocating*!' I think so far, I've been happy to talk about my Leukaemia as it's all new stuff, but I've arrived at a similar point (and I also don't see the point of people having *their* lives blighted with all this thought).

Macmillan Nurses produced a book about what to say to cancer patients. The trouble is only patients read it. They made this point too. Also they suggest not telling stories of other people with cancer. In the last 2 days I've had a tale forwarded to me with the line, 'There's no pain like cancer pain' (gee thanks – I'm sure tooth ache is a good rival: pain is pain) and another friend telling me *I'm lucky* because 2 other friends of hers with Leukaemia have died. Besides, unless anyone can tell me a story about someone with my AML with the same factor of 5 – and I'm sure no one can – then I'm really no more interested than the average person.

Yes I'm sure the approximately 50 folk who receive this email across the globe (along with a similar number of those it gets forwarded to) can see I'm back to my usual 'tell it like it is' self – but imagine if just 10% of that 100 think that their stories are what you need! I have to say that male friends have been the ones who have left it to the doctors *to 'fix me'*. Thanks guys. Also I see now the mistakes I have made in the past with others.

Prayers for all to go smoothly however would be appreciated. In some ways I've had a lot of bad luck in hospital so far – the burn on my arm, the line that fell in my heart and the nerve damage. However, when I've said this to 2 different friends, they both gave the same reply – '*Think about the good luck of having a 10/10 match donor*!' And of course, they are right. Also the heart monitor showed my heart to be OK!!! The nerve damage may repair itself given time. But I am disappointed I have to have the same chemo again with this possible side effect. Please pray for no more damage! Lastly on the positive side, my sister has been able to relocate the family holiday to August so there's now a chance I'll be present.

I hope I haven't offended anyone in this email. I know it's hard to get it right – too much or not enough – but I do know there's a lot of love out there for me,

Hazel

Friends 34

Dear All,

Loud music drifted up to me this morning from outside my room in Barts – it was the London Marathon passing St. Paul's.

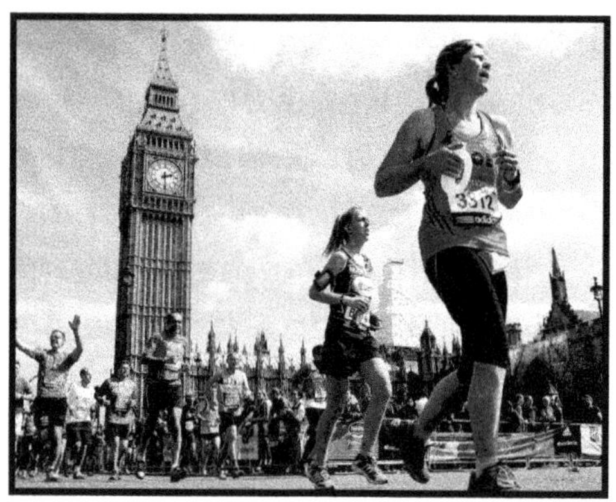

2015: those marathon runners at Big Ben.

Inside the room we are on a marathon of our own – 24 tablets & 7 drips yesterday and again today.

My Consultant asked how I was when I arrived. 'Fine,' I replied, 'It's you who's going to make me feel ill!' (It was great to be free to enjoy a couple of weeks of feeling really fit and like my old self before arriving).

They are now taking me down in preparation for hopefully installing someone else's immune system on Wednesday. By the way this does not involve an operating theatre as one friend had the impression – I just lie in my bed, while the stem cells (that arrive frozen) are put into like a fish tank to whoosh around to separate, then they have a 20min window before they die off, to pump them into me with a large injection needle.

The donor is male and 'old!' (as my Consultant exclaimed). I think 46 is the cut off age for going on the Anthony Nolan register although one would remain on it for some years afterwards. Thank God for this kind person who will experience some discomfort at having the cells removed from his larger bones in return for no reward. In time I will be allowed to send a message.

On my side it will be 'rescue by the colonials' this time. I am a state whose security has failed [to stop adolescent white cells leaving the bone prematurely when they *don't know* how to do their job of fighting infections & instead spend their time proliferating wildly]. The entry of a colonial power needs to be welcomed, even though they are there *to take over* and dwell, not give temporary help and hope you'll be ok when they leave (like chemo). I must *welcome* them simply because I recognise I cannot do the job of dealing with Leukaemia cells myself. This is hard for *anybody* to do ('*I'm all right, don't need your help*').

To me the only experience I can liken it to is handing over my life to God when I was 19 when I recognised that I couldn't do the job of living a good life myself. I *allowed* the washing away of all *shortcomings* (past, present & future) by the blood of *Jesus*. (As you all know only too well knowing me, this doesn't *force* you into *good behaviour* as ISIS and the Puritans before them did – without changing the human heart: I still make bad choices which hurt others, but when you choose the opposite, the power & opportunity come.)

When I first arrived in a ward at Barts late at night way back in October, there were neither staff nor patients to be seen – then through a long narrow window I saw 2 men in pyjamas who had lost their hair, staring out; where the hell have I arrived I thought – Belsen? Here I have a nice room on my own as we all do, but now we are even more isolated as all patients have an anti-chamber to enter through (bit like Tutankhamen's tomb), so that even if you look in a window you can't see anybody. After 3 days, I saw 2 men in the dayroom.

However in walking the corridors, I do see visitors. I talk particularly to the sister of Mohammed, a man in his 20s. The extended family usually gather attentively outside his room, and I have become friendly with them all. He has had 2 transplants from a sibling. Neither has prevented its return in the long run and he is now on pain management. (BT are wrong – it isn't always 'good to talk'!)

Another girl had appendicitis in the middle of chemo treatment (they don't even like you having dental treatment till you've recovered, let alone going under the knife!) and I thought I'd been unlucky!

Must rush now, Coronation Street on at 9 every day this week . . .

Friends 35

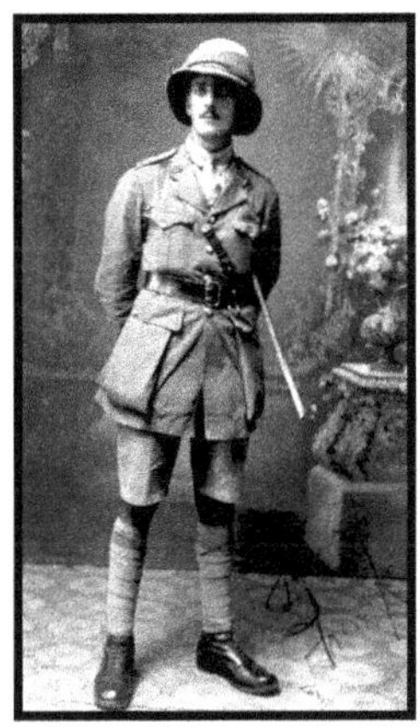

'The colonials have arrived!'

Dear Friends, etc.,

A week since the transplant so an update:

On DAY ZERO, as the Anthony Nolan Trust call it, I was very calm – I awoke from a dream where one of the property programme presenters achieved an *incredible* long jump! (She's a pretty blonde, but with very short legs actually.)

Problem with courier made the stem cell arrival late, so I phoned my bank to enquire about interest for my tax returns, as you do. To 'Have a nice afternoon!' I replied that I was having a bone marrow transplant. A pause. Time to consider professional etiquette – then the response came, 'I had one when I was 2'. A moment of 'God-incidence' hit us both.

To those who read carefully, you will recall the transplant is *not* about fighting and being strong, but about allowing. My recent psalm referred back to the incident where one of the Kings was told '*You will not have to fight this battle. Take up your positions; stand firm and see the deliverance the Lord will give you*'. Well, my position was to lie on the bed, while the nurse took half an hour to find a vein large enough to take the tube; then in the presence of the nurse and a friend of mine, the infusion took around another half hour. Both of these men have a lovely tranquil spirit. The donor must have given the cells that morning, for they arrived fresh (resembling homemade tomato soup, not that I'd be an expert in that), so no need for fish tank & whooshing, just a big drip.

A week on, the message is: 'All Quiet on the Western Front!' I feel *fine* – apart from when I have to take 15 tablets at a time and then eat fish & cold chips! Those stem cells will take another week to all find their way to the bigger bones and take up their positions and effect changes. The guy who runs a Friday vegetable stall in my parents' village asked, '*How do they know* where to go?' I shall refer his question to the Professor on his next round (I *suspect* they go everywhere looking for the best fit).

The Professor enjoyed my colonial analogy and entered my room with 'The colonials have arrived!' There will hopefully be minor skirmishes along the way (Graft-versus-Host disease is actually *necessary* to show the new immune system can fight the Leukaemia if it returns). Strangely for an uprising, the *date* of the major rebellion is *known*. It is on DAY 100 which will be early September. That is when the helpful *suppression* of my old immune system is *removed*. Released from house arrest, the old will see the new as the foreign body &

vice-versa. A fight will ensue. Perhaps we could call it 'The 100 Day War'. I've been fascinated to read the blog of a young Jewish New Yorker who had my same AML cancer. The treatments were virtually identical along with his similar thoughts. He didn't make it to Day 100 but he's a good writer and so it's worth looking at (note US spelling): survivingLeukaemia.wordpress.com.

Well, as the song goes 'there could be trouble ahead'. But let's hope we can face it & come out dancing (*corny* or what!). Should this present 'good behaviour' continue however, I could be out in 7 days, the doctor said.

The letter at the end of this, is what I handwrote anonymously to my donor, which I'm allowed to send. In 2 years we are able to meet, if he's interested & I'm still around. I've been a busy little bee submitting my tax form 10 months early, calculating the price increases for my business for next term and catching up on 11 months of personal accounts. I've also been planning my funeral with performances (sorry no Egyptian music & dance this time). I got quite carried away with it and found myself wishing it could be soon!! Lol.

I liaised with a friend over the funeral plans. She is in the half of the world who believe (& can never be persuaded by the rest of us who think otherwise) that *mention* of something makes it *more likely* to occur – and suggested the format could be used for my *marriage* (no candidate so far, but for those of you who are in that half, do, do *mention* it.) I thought it an excellent idea but said we may have to leave out the Treorchy Cemetery bit.

This is such a strange ward with its anti-chambers isolating us. I have seen 4 other patients now – although 8 others are said to exist. Last Wednesday's Breakfast Club there was only 1 other 'walking wounded' present, so they had to bus in some nurses. Let's go now to avoid the crush for the croissants. Later, Jayne my sister visiting from Wales for 3 days, is bringing in a lunchtime Carluccio's take-away. What a good day for me, with an appetite such as I've never had in my life. For any who are fasting along with praying for me – permission to eat!

Hazel

Dear Donor

Today I received your stem cells. What can I say, except 'Thank You'. I hope the process was not too painful or inconvenient. I'm grateful you followed through on your intention.

I expect you wonder where they've ended up! Well in a 63-year-old woman with Leukaemia. After feeling tired on and off for a year, I went from one day teaching dance in a Primary School, to A&E the next.

Thus started my journey with Leukaemia last October, and I've spent most of the time since then in hospital - having never been admitted in my life. I had 3 lots of chemo but mine is a type of Leukaemia that likes to come back. My own immune system turns out to be inadequate - so I'm trying out yours!

My ambitions for living include looking after my elderly parents - eventually burying them (rather than have them bury me) - and to finish my autobiography for I've had an interesting life and travelled much.

Thank you once more for your part in blessing my family and large circle of friends by providing an opportunity to extend my life. May you and yours be blessed in return,

Your Recipient

Friends 36

Wrote this last Wednesday, but no WiFi to send it:

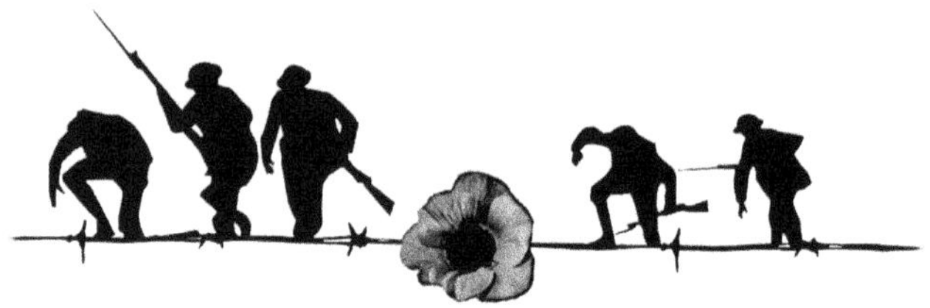

Position as of today is that I'm still in hospital waiting for that 0.5. Amusing myself writing my funeral leaflet now (well someone's got to do it & this way I get to have my favourite songs & pictures). Hopefully it will need a good deal of updating by the time I actually die, but the point is if you get sick you may not be well enough to bother – the patient Mohammed, drove himself here; tragically he is now too ill to be driven home to die. From the aging Rasta on one side of my wall to this young Bengali, nothing joins us together except the illness & our common humanity.

Now a few days later, I'm writing this after crying a few tears, tears of relief. I just held in my hand the evidence that the new stem cells are working; a white piece of paper with my blood counts on. Theory is all well & good, but the reality is proved *here*.

Today marks 2 weeks since the transplant, and the estimated time it would take for the stem cells to arrive in the marrow. Red and white cells are leaping up, likewise platelets. Those all-important neutrophils that control infection reappeared – currently 0.2 (normal level 2 to 7): 0.5 and I can go home. We have bought time, & ultimately time is all any of us has. Without treatment, I may not even have seen 2015.

As Churchill said though: 'This is not the end. This is not even the beginning of the end. But it *is* the end of the beginning'. From here the stem cells will have to:

- Deal with any infections, hopefully not meeting any unmatched to its strength.

- Fight my old immune system when it is released in September.

- Ultimately fight the return of Leukaemia.

Power to its elbow!

Another doctor said stem cell use will become *very common* (good job I got in early then). I suggested he set up shop next to the tattoo parlour. I took his praise about how well I'd come through the chemo & the transplant: from his tone I suspected that he himself would not have given me the full treatment. Later I wondered what exactly *I had done* – when I met him in the corridor, I told him that what I hadn't said was that a lot of people were praying for me: 'Tell them they've done well' was his curt reply.

I *feel* fit too, cycling a mile on the exercise bike in only 8.4 min (lol). I dread the return of the physiotherapist though; I haven't had any time to do her exercises. However, there was no getting away from the large Polish assistant who breezed into my room, put The Wombles Song on her phone, and said '*Now* – we will DANCE!' It was up out of bed we go, holding hands and doing twirls. I dare say it wouldn't suit some.

It's been a good thing not having a TV in the room; in which case I would only have lived life in the intervals between my programmes. Instead, I've been finishing accounts, choreographing a dance for church, and turning the 'Letter to my Donor' into a song! Tamara, my friend I knew in New York, in reply to my last email, said that her sister *specialises* in singing songs about the Big C. I gave permission for her to do whatever she wanted, and also set to myself – composing to the tune of 'Camp Granada' (Hello Muddah, Hello Faddah)! Next time you are over The Pond, perhaps you'll hear it in a Greenwich Village folk club.

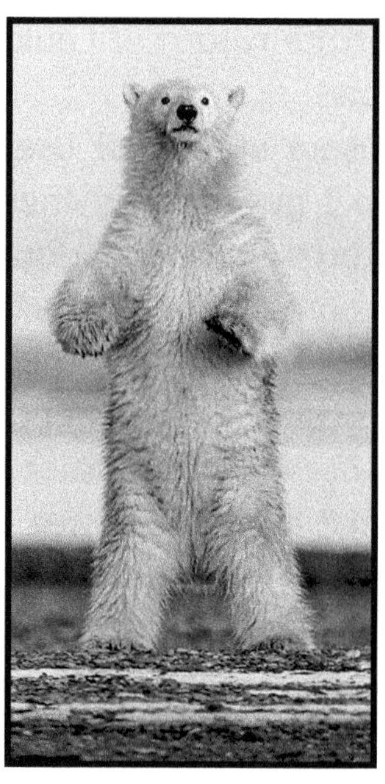

So, it looks like I will be out very shortly. I have faced the polar bear – for those of you I shared my dream with. When my 3rd chemo was ending, I was given a book to read about the forthcoming transplant. In the library you could probably find it under Horror Stories, for there is *nothing* positive in that book. The question one is left with is '*Why the Hell would anyone have this done*?' Making the mistake of reading it late at night, I fell asleep and awoke in terror after seeing a HUGE white polar bear standing before me.

I slept again and dreamed that the bear, now a lot smaller, was sleeping at the far side of my bed. I reached out my hand to stroke him and the fur was as baby-soft as my friend Terri's new hair that she had asked me to feel that morning. What was surprising was how quickly I went from one scenario to the other.

Yes, home from the Arctic soon, but you never know what'll happen next here: the door opens and a 6hr magnesium drip suddenly arrives. I *already* take 4 magnesium tablets a day! *It's a good job it's just a trace element*, was my comment. Actually, the serious point is that the medical profession *can* overdose you, as with my father who spent an agonising 3 weeks in hospital with an overdose of calcium. When he left, the doctor said to me that *that* level of calcium 'was not thought to be consistent with life'. It took a while to sink in. He hadn't said '*health*' but '*life*'.

So, life to you all – I shall be sharing a toast with my lodgers at home soon; Phil bought the champagne in France in readiness.

L'chaim! (To Life: Hebrew)

Hazel

Friends 37

Three weeks since the transplant, I'm out of hospital and still feeling fine!

You know when back in April, my dedicated nurse told me: 'Some people having a transplant have no symptoms at all' – it was like someone announcing to your class that there'd be a new hockey team; you just knew *that you* were not going to be in it. But by the grace of God, it was me this time!

At home, I'm enjoying simple pleasures like being able to open the window and to feel the breeze. Despite hoping to be less manic, from the hospital I went to my friend David's*, and we enjoyed recording the song I'd written after a half-hour practice. Couldn't wait to get it right as his baby had to go to bed & my throat was getting more & more sore. It turned out a bit spoof (although my thanks to the donor are profound), but it may cheer some poor soul facing the big bear to think 'Well she's still standing there 3 weeks on (& maybe she was that mad before anyway)'. See it on:
https://www.youtube.com/watch?v=NAfN4b2iiLk

I hope to be in Wales later this week but can't go for long from London because suppressants have to be finely tuned (the level is toxic at first). I say 'I hope' because this will be the new Hazel – unreliable.

- Any arrangement I make may have to be cancelled at short notice due to health.
- 2ndly I am not allowed crowds; but am trying to

be creative going to the open-air theatre & sitting on the end of the row!

- 3rdly I have to take care around children. If any of yours develop chickenpox, measles etc *after* my visit, kindly let me know as I have to inform the hospital.
- 4thly please help me to stay healthy by not hugging or kissing.

Although the journey's not over, I imagine emails from me will decrease. Thanks for sharing the ride.

Hazel

**David Morris, the laconic guitarist, played a rather different role in the 1990's. In the 2½ year McLibel trial (the longest in English history) along with his co-defendant, and with no law training but a host of global support, David fought the giant McDonalds. Name dropping? Of course, what's the point of having famous friends?*

Friends 38

Dear Friends,

Well that was a good long rest from me, wasn't it? But lots are asking for an update so here it is. However, if you feel satisfied with the story ending as it was, do tell me & I'll unsubscribe.

I am well; I go to the hospital now every other week and they are pleased with me thus far. I have energy every day, but at some point it's like someone has pulled my battery out and I want to sleep. I managed the family holiday in Somerset, and a short break away with a friend, but I envy others going abroad – perhaps in times past they envied me?

Anyway, those who've seen me say I look better than before I went ill – mostly due to the grey hair which seems to suit me (it's come back straight!) I'm about to have my first haircut. Sunday I went to the Brian Adams/Rod Stewart concert in Hyde Park! So me and Rod looked

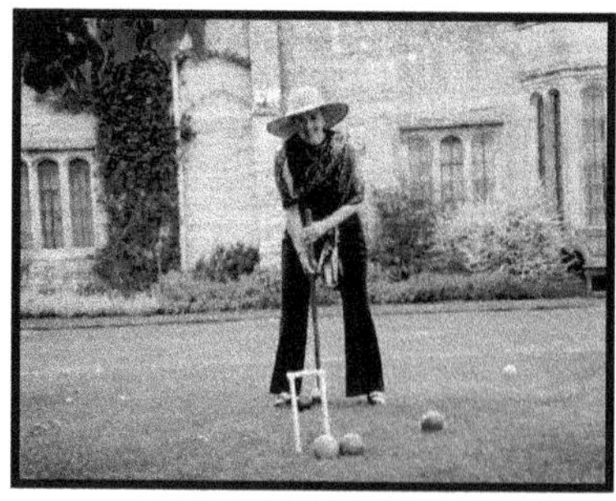

Somerset: anyone for croquet?

good – not too sure about the crowds of *elderly* people who knew all the words to the Brian Adams songs (I'm *too* old to know them myself).

However I'm not out of the woods. The odds of living for 5 years (is that counting the one I've had?) has only just swung *in my favour* (it was something like 1 in 6 last October). Because of the transplant, I now have a 50% chance of making it; and my Consultant and I reckoned that we could add 5% to that, out of the 10% chance of dying from the transplant – due to the fact of not having done so yet. But at the end of the day (or rather the 5 years) you either 100% make it or 100% don't.

Yes, ten days ago, we passed the marker point of 100 days after the transplant! The significance of this is that my original immune system now has to be gradually allowed to *re-emerge*. Thus the medication suppressing it is being reduced. When my old immune system returns it will ask 'Who are you?' to the new donor one – who will be asking the same question back! A fight will ensue: the Battle of 'Graft-versus-Host disease'. Some of us have been here before & will see a parallel with Paul's description of the 'old man' *in our nature*, & the incoming 'new man' rendering the old powerless (in his letter to the people in Rome).

If there is no evidence of a fight, the doctors will not be happy, as the fight is necessary for the new immune system to cut its teeth on, for when/if it has to fight the return of Leukaemia. If the fight is too severe, it's another route of demise! So I literally have to *hope* for *somewhat* of a fight, which could take many forms.

At present I am vulnerable also to all disease as my childhood inoculations were knocked out by the transplant. I'm supposed to avoid crowds; open air events are fine, but I guess there won't be too many more of those as the weather turns. I've had my first injection of 15 this year. The live MMR injection will be in 2 years.

Last time we checked my blood group hadn't changed, but the donor has been busy making some other positive changes – the rare *mf* skin condition I already had, has so far not been seen since the transplant (a transplant was a treatment for it but I'd never have been serious enough to have that risk prescribed).

A few years ago I had a dear friend who had Leukaemia and lived for a few years. When she died I said to her son, 'But I thought she was *all right*!' He replied that she *was* all right *until she wasn't*. That sums up the situation really. Anyway I'm thankful for the time that the girl's all right.

Regards,
Hazel

Friends 39

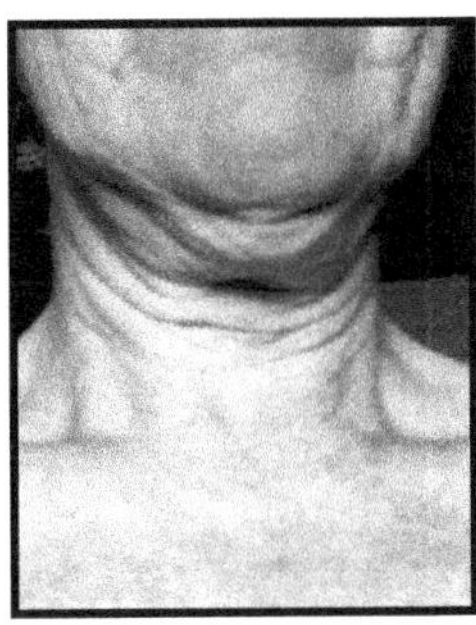

That's what I call a rash! Consultant remarked last time.

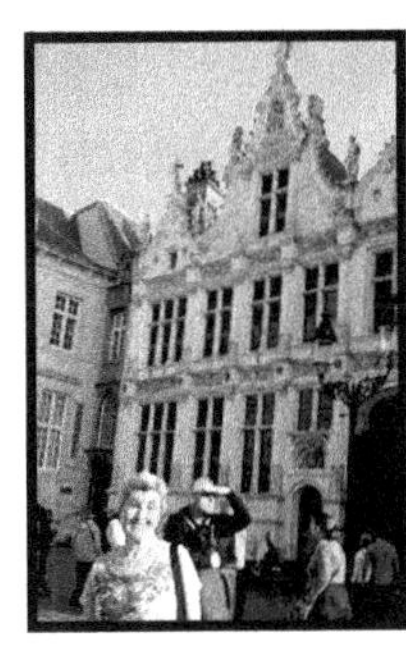

Consultant now gave the OK for me to travel.

Dear All,

Some folk have been wondering and the answer is I've been *extremely well* since I last wrote – even to the point of managing 4 days in Brugge on my own (twice as long as the average tourist!)

I won't go over all of the anticipated fight between my 2 immune systems – it's there on Friends 38 sent 15th Sept. What I didn't realise *at that time*, is that it would only be likely to happen after *today's* further reduction in the medication keeping my old immune system out of the way. So thanks for any prayers sent aforetime.

It's like sitting tight waiting for an enemy to arrive & battle commence, except that the enemy is within – the immune system I was born with is now being allowed to stagger out, and fight the new immune system. This donor immune system is running the show and doing very well too. It saw off my recent sore throat (last year's failure to end 5 weeks of laryngitis was what led to the discovery of Leukaemia) & stopped me getting a cold from Mum while staying in a caravan with them. (I've also had 6 of my 12 childhood injections that have to be reinstated this year – now look at kids as slightly less potentially lethal.)

The result will be the permanent deletion as the Consultant put it (*death* to the rest of us) of the old system, hopefully without the battle giving *me* a 'new address' too. The latter is one of the cards on the table, but the peaceful co-existence of the 2 systems, which some have wished for me, is *not* an option.

The evidence of the fight that the Consultant needs to see, can come in a variety of forms; I'm hoping for a rash as I've had 3 horrific ones this year, and life goes on. However, I was slightly unnerved by meeting a chap at my last appointment who'd had his transplant 16 months before me, both of us from a stranger (there's less reaction if from a sibling). He had to go back in for 2 months, now has permanent damage to his gut, mouth & skin, and has had to return to the suppressants. Presumably he'll have to have another try later. I'm hoping for a better outcome!!

I'm encouraged by remembering how afraid I was before the transplant (the polar bear nightmare) which turned out in my case to be a walk in the park rather than the Arctic. Also, I'm hoping that there's an algorithm set up in me (no I don't really understand the word either, just trying it out) whereby, because I 'have previous' in the battle between the old nature and the new one *in my spirit*, my *body* will go with the pattern sometimes set & defer to the better one.

So here's to hope!

Hazel

Friends 40

Dear Friends,

What! You again! – In my defence, I note only 2 of these emails from me in the last 6 months.

This is because THE HEADLINES have been good:

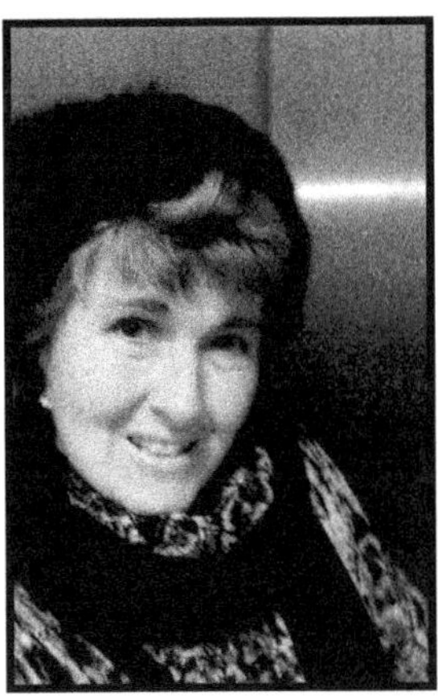

Me looking Russian: another selfie!

- Now 1 YEAR this month since in remission (although I had to have another course of the strong chemo to back it up after that time, along with the transplant, so *it doesn't seem* that long).

- My blood counts have gone up each time they're tested. I'm on the normal scale for fighting infection – towards the lower end, but my immune system saw off my first cold without it developing into worse.

- Today I celebrate being 64, when without treatment I

would have been unlikely to have seen 63 (not travelling to Wales but at least not in hosp).

The SMALL PRINT however has been pretty miserable as I've been going through the Graft-versus-Host stage, expected after my old immune system was let out as the suppression was reduced.

A number of areas have been chosen battle sites, but my mouth has given the most trouble. I was in Wales for 4 weeks over Christmas and it was a bit scary to cope with up to 4 different fungus/infections, when so far from Barts Hosp. Since those passed, I've had areas of mouth ulcer – about the most painful thing in the whole illness! I'm now on steroids and can eat soft food.

Actually the 'fight' metaphors useful in the past are now, according to my Consultant, to be seen as stages in a relationship:

The period after the transplant was like an *early stage* of a relationship, when the *similarities* between 2 persons, is apparent (after all, the *outside* of the donor's cells were a 10/10 match with mine).

Now with the reduction in the suppressant, the real me is emerging and the new guy is shocked at the *differences* – after all I am non-related, female and a polar-opposite blood group (the reaction would be worse if I was a man having a woman taking over apparently). The new guy is therefore attacking *me*.

We have to move to a 3rd stage the Consultant said, where he learns to *tolerate* me.

Boy does this put me off the thought of ever getting married! Think I'll stick to 'the road less trod'.

Hopefully, this *may be* the only incidence of the fight I'll experience, or it may grumble on for up to 2yrs. I have ambitions this year to go on a walking holiday in Italy, and a wedding I'm invited to in Ethiopia. We'll have to wait to see how things go though.

But remember, the HEADLINES are good!

I amused myself on the weekend by reading all of the previous 39 emails! They weren't at times as lucid as I imagined, but it was interesting to view the journey & at times to see how little I realised was still ahead.

Best wishes to all,

Hazel

Friends 41

Dear Friends, etc.

Last week it was 'World Cancer Day' I noted as I crossed London to attend a travel exhibition. In honour I am bringing out the 'Boxed Set' of my 40 emails to Friends – the attached chapter which combines them neatly forming part of my autobiography. It will be of interest to the under-occupied, also those of you who pointed out you missed some emails – and with the frustrating lack of Wi-Fi in hospital I never got round to filling you in using the dongle.

Thanks for your support everyone (& especially to Barts) – I am now finding pleasure in the days. Last week I was energised by doing a dance day in a school for one of the dancers who was ill! I have booked a

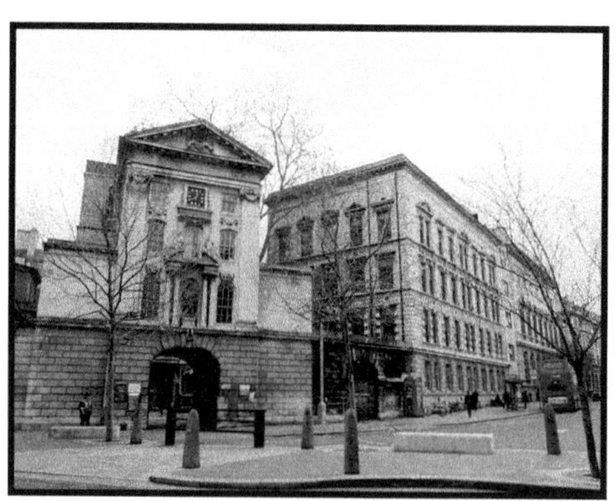

The 1702 gate
Barts survived the Fire of London
& much of the Blitz.

walking holiday in Italy next month, made arrangements leading to attending a wedding in Ethiopia in May, and bought my cards for next Christmas. (I can't have live injections until May '17, so if Yellow Fever gets me, the last biography chapter will be 'And they buried her in Abyssinia': which will add a certain air of romance.)

I haven't come out unscathed (*in fact have not come out yet, as had to up the suppressant again this week – but we're sniffing the air of freedom*). There remains damage to leg nerves from one of the 6 types of chemo used and I have to take into account I'm less stable on my feet. Mouth problems seem to have eroded gum and I suspect teeth are also less stable now. But the 3rd degree chemo burn in my arm is almost negligible – doctors can cut out, join, and kill, but only God can actually heal.

What really happened to me? I've got more of a handle on it now:

1. Sometime in 2013 *one* stem cell (a baby cell) decided *not* to grow up, develop into a cell that has a job, work and then die. (No doubt these things are happening to us all on a daily basis, but this, unlike other changes, passed under my radar – no one else was responsible). The cells multiplied, left the Nursery of the bone marrow and reproduced wildly, even crowding out cells that were faithfully doing their job in my blood. Thus the tiredness I noticed for a year leading to the inability to fight laryngitis. [Later the parallel posed itself with those rejecting the quiet work & faith of their parents' generation, attracting other young recruits and making a bid for immortality in battle.]

2. By the time I presented myself to A&E in Oct '14 I couldn't make it to the bus stop home (though I had

managed to lead a dance day in the Midlands the day before!) One look at my blood sent the doctor out of A&E to find me (learn folk, I should have had a blood test before this).

3. Without the availability of chemo and being judged fit enough to have it at 62 (my heart was good and the laryngitis had not weakened me too much), I would have been dead for a year now.

4. I failed the first bout of chemo & turned out to have had a chromosome change after all. After Consultants deciding I *could* face 2 courses of stronger chemo, the cancer was dead but I had an 85% chance of it returning.

5. With the donor stem cell transplant in May I am down to a 33% chance of the Leukaemia returning in the next 5 years – usually in first 2 (I've had 1!). If it doesn't, they term it 'a cure'.

So what am I left with for future aspirations?

Talking about illness a lot less I jolly well hope & getting on with having plans while knowing the saying (you may too): 'Man proposes: God disposes'. But I prefer to put it more positively, 'For me to live is Christ: to die is gain' (course St Paul said that first), which is the same as I felt 16 months ago.

Many years back I decided that if serious illness came *my* way, I wouldn't be *desperate* for healing. I'd simply ask for it and have a preference to live. I found that very relaxing when the day came that I *was* diagnosed. Then in the physical process that followed there *was* fighting, but I felt I myself was allowing & observing it, in the battlefield of my body – at times suffering from its fall-out (without pain thankfully – that *definitely* would have shown a different me).

What about you lot?

– Did any of you sign up as blood donors? One day I needed 3 pints! Or as stem cell donors? (Isn't it great news that on Tuesday the Leukaemia patient who is half Italian & half Thai found a donor!!)

– Have you signed the petition against eroding the National Health Service, or watched the film:
www.selloff.org.uk
You could forward this.

Now some folk think Hazel *doesn't like* men: not so (although just as a teacher friend said about children – '*they're ok but I couldn't eat a whole one*'). 2 men have now saved my life!

- The anonymous donor with his stem cells which have been enthusiastic in their purpose of entering my blood *to work*, then *die* (at first trying to kill me off as well!)

- Jesus with *his* blood rebooting me in the sight of God, *to co-operate together* here, and *live* forever (not in *this* world as that baby stem cell tried to do in *his* bid for immortality)

I saw a T-shirt picturing a cross once with the slogan: 'Body piercing saved my life'.

I can add, 'twice'.

Cheers,

Hazel

(If you think this could help someone you know, feel free to fwd – or if you have ideas on how to put before a larger audience, let me know bearing in mind I'm too old & busy for Twitter, Facebook, Instagram, etc.)

Friends 42

Or 'Will this woman never stop talking?'

If you wish to forward the 'Boxed Set' & haven't yet done so, kindly use this version. My Consultant suggested sending it to a patients' website also.

Those of a nervous disposition may like to avoid the photos provided of me ill – it could have been worse, I left out the 'hairy black tongue' one!

Fabulous news today in the press – the *SAS version* of rescue for Leukaemia I'd looked towards, targeting only cancer cells, has been developed, and first trials are coming up with huge success on a group of terminal cases. I dare say it will be some time down the line for *all*.

In contrast, the *rescue by the Russians* version I had, the chemo targeting all fast-growing cells in the body, is typified today by news of their bombing of hospitals & schools in Syria. I visited Syria some years ago and was impressed not only by the amazing medieval cities but by the kindness of the people towards me. (Recently I wrote of one of these acts in a letter to *The Metro* alongside their current plight, and a Reader replied he'd burst into tears on a crowded train!)

Today also came the reality check of buying travel insurance for a week in Italy – unfortunately my walking holiday next month want a*ll medical conditions* covered. Most companies would not cover me; none would offer Annual Insurance. These are *the people who know* – at a

1 out of 3 chance of not surviving, the players of Russian roulette would also be thin on the ground. Eventually I got insurance for just under £200 for the *week*! (A friend's was £110 for the *year* with the Americas included.)

On the other hand, today I had a great day – a bird walk in the forest with my great niece (no bird was spotted due to being with a group of children, but I refrained from doing my school teacher bit), and precious time spent with my parents.

Regards,
Hazel

Friends 43

Dear All,

Waking up to the sound of the crashing waves (OK actually a text message woke me at 9.30) . . . but I *am* by the sea in the caravan in West Wales on my own, for a 'writing week'. Well, that autobiography was one of the reasons I hoped to go on living and I've done precious little to further it in the months since, due partly to lack of energy some days, as still clearing poisons from the body perhaps – did you hear recently that chemo is developed from Mustard Gas? And then there's the time spent with hospital visits, family, friends, the dance business (*yes we know, but you're lazy too, Hazel*). This is the 4th day & not started writing yet, but for it to hold together I need to re-read what I've written, some of it over 10 years ago.

I'm diverting to writing this brief general email to mark 2 YEARS TODAY since I found myself on a trolley in the store cupboard of my local hospital (no I assured them, I didn't mind – anywhere in the hospital being better than anywhere outside it); then that late night transfer to Barts with no staff on the ward desk and the ambulance men not knowing what to do – resulting in me going off looking for someone to admit me, wondering as I passed Belsen-like patients whether I would soon be resembling them.

Still coming to terms with it all, I was admitted with what I now believe to have been perhaps less than a 10% chance of survival due to age & what transpired to be the worst category of chromosome change. But those cells are all gone now with the Leukaemia, and my new immune system is driving off even potential colds! There is also no sign of the previous 'incurable' condition I had.

In the medical world, it's wonderful that not only are those targeted treatments being worked on – '*like a sniper selecting precisely who to take out*' (their words) – but also immunotherapies switching on our own defences against cancer, '*acting like the Black Ops of cancer treatment*'. In point of fact, a guy from my church has had the latter this autumn! Strange how the battle for Mosul dominates news today, reminding me of how the battle for Kobane seemed to me to parallel the medical profession's fight for my life.

My emails from that time continue to bring feedback, even last week a young friend was telling me how much she looked forward to my emails from hospital. I'm glad I wasn't one of those miserable patients, & gave folk enjoyment, besides shock & concern. I've wondered since if thinking they'd never see me again motivated some of my hospital visitors. I still visit Barts every 5 weeks, they say I'll never be discharged (I guess that's so long as there's an NHS!)

Anyway, just to let you know *I'm well*. After a necessary, but long period of Graft-versus-Host problems, the suppressant is being reduced. (It was the suppressant which killed the face-transplant person recently you may have heard – gosh, so many things that could kill you!) Having survived the process – including 4 types of Superbugs – besides possible skirmishes, we now have to survive the peace.

After Ethiopia this year, I have big travel plans for next year in place. If they are God's will, they will be fulfilled.

Regards,
Hazel

Life after the War

Much time has now passed since these dispatches and I will fill in the gap:

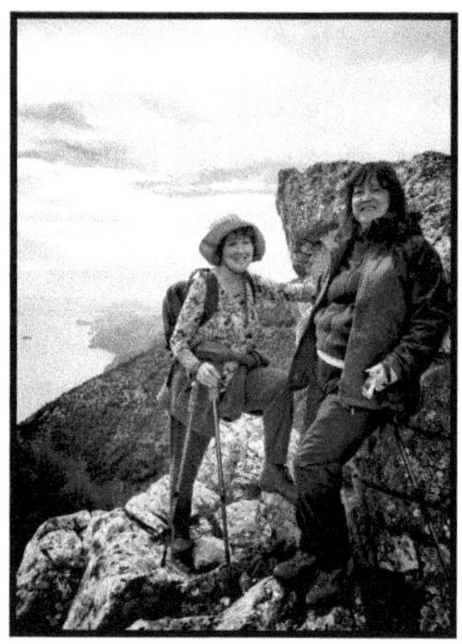

I survived that walking holiday on the Amalfi 'coast', using walking poles to aid my legs lacking balance (unfortunately no one had told me that we were situated halfway up a mountain with walks mainly being up or down it). It was particularly fulfilling as it was with Norah, the friend I'd done so badly at walking with in Bara. The others in the group gave me a clap at the end, and I hadn't *seriously* held them up either.

As with my earlier trip to Brugge where I was looking forward to meeting *new* people, particularly people who didn't know me as 'ill', I actually found myself talking about my recent illness with the other walkers. It was not something to be ignored by me, or hidden from others; it was part of who I now was.

'If you're trying to make me feel jealous, you're succeeding!' I had written from my hospital bed to Jo on her emails from Ethiopia and Zanzibar. We'd taught together in Nigeria, and now both of those locations were within reach of where she was working in Tanzania. But shortly – and strangely – I had the privilege of going to both Ethiopia and Zanzibar myself!

It was out of the blue that a Hungarian friend invited me to attend her son's wedding in Ethiopia. I laughed at first – but I not only went but left the wedding group after a week and travelled alone to the north, to see the amazing churches dug down into the rock surface. It was a risk, but the first person I met on arriving at the small hotel was an American nurse who had worked with Leukaemia patients. He and his Ethiopian wife offered to help me clamber along the wet rocks to enter the churches. Can you believe it?

The next year I hankered after attending that African Music Festival in Zanzibar, but didn't want to be presumptuous. Within a few days, my neighbour in London declared, 'I'm going to Zanzibar!' Now when did you ever hear someone say that? I took it as a Yes for my journey, and we saw each other a few times in the fantastic festival. I then journeyed on to the mainland of Tanzania to stay with the friend who had made me so jealous!

A dance holiday in Andalucia followed – the pace was leisurely and again I was able to keep up. Back in the UK Linda, my dance partner, and I performed twice in a small show – after the first, I went straight to A&E as Graft-versus-Host had begun in my lungs. I hadn't known what was wrong, but 3 min into my dance, it seemed *impossible* to

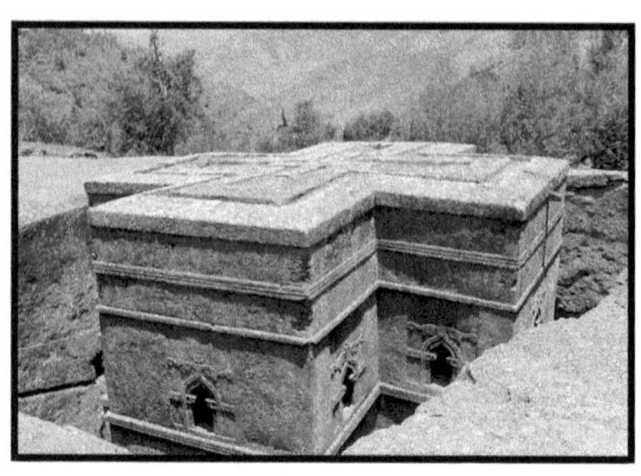

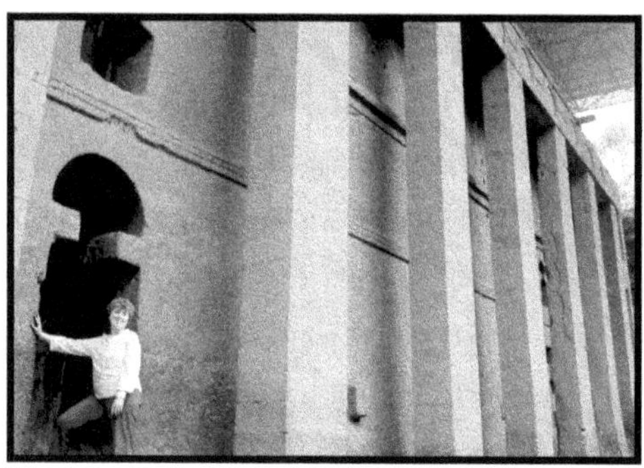

go on. Unfortunately the dance was 5 min long! (With 70 pairs of eyes on me, I just moved on the spot, and somehow fudged it). At my lowest, I could only even *walk* for 2 min, but after a course of steroids, the next year's performance was less of a drama.

Apart from continuing my business running workshops in schools with the drummer by hiring other dancers as and when, and doing the admin, I also took on some of the dance bookings myself – despite lungs having some permanent damage. Two and a half years after suddenly ringing my drummer to say I couldn't attend the booking in 2 days as I was in hospital for 'a month' ('Blimey, what's wrong with you?'), I passed the baton on to him and retired.

Two years after the Anthony Nolan Foundation ar-

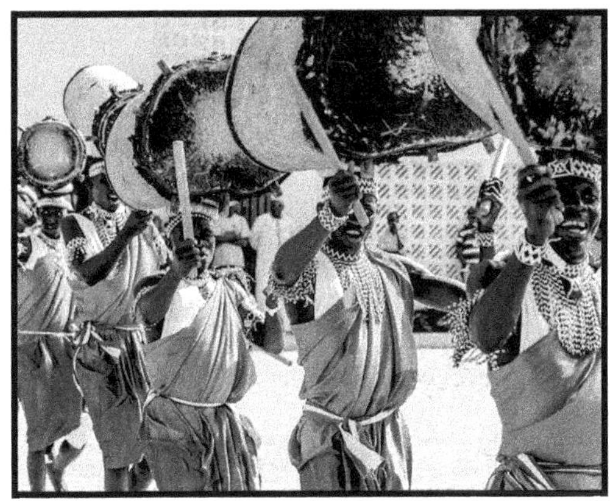

Festival.

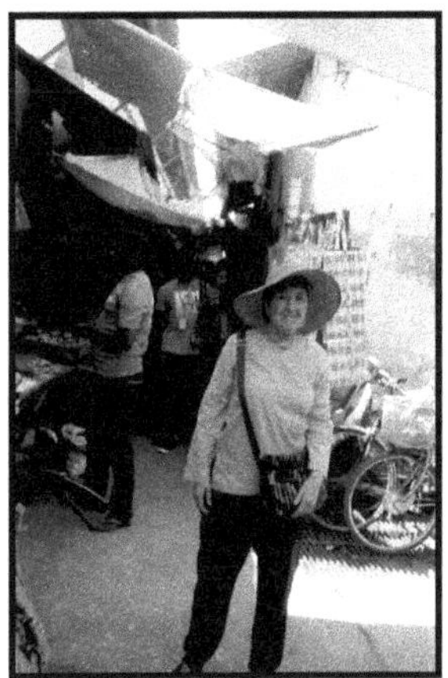

Braving Stone Town Market, Zanzibar.

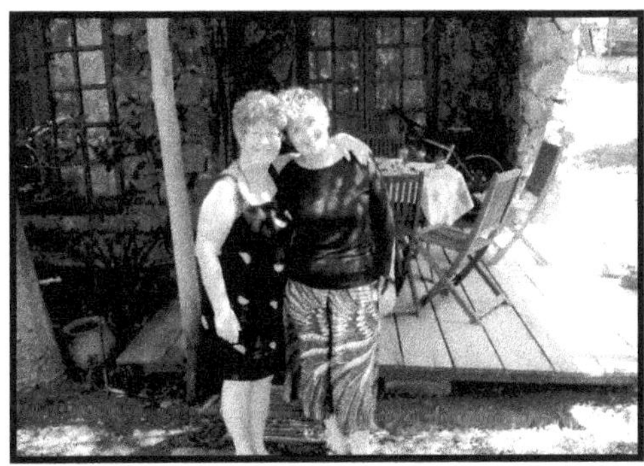

With that friend Jo!

ranged my transplant, it was possible to meet my donor. I wrote again but he never replied. Funnily enough, one day when I was on a journey back to Wales with a guy from the RAC in a pick-up truck (my car loaded on the back), in the course of the long conversation, he mentioned that *he'd* been a donor and never heard from the recipient. He took it when I gave him my thanks in place of what he had not received.

The outside of my eyes is now dried up by Graft-versus-Host (I wonder if the other 10/10 donor match might have been kinder to me, while still doing his main job of keeping away Leukaemia?) I have now been granted daily capsules of serum from blood donors, which hydrate better than other eye drops, to try out: more good people to thank. I *was* a blood donor myself. On receiving my 15th pint of blood, I was discouraged – on balance I would now be a *recipient*, and I stopped a strict count after that.

While a young blood donor, I had asked to register as a bone marrow donor. 'You don't want to do that: it's painful' said the woman at the session. I was a stranger to pain . . . and Reader, imagine . . . I walked away.

Appointments at Barts – which is apparently Britain's oldest continuous hospital on one site – although now down to 3 monthly, mostly with the very amicable Dr Oakervee, were for a time multitude: I was indeed on a short leash! Septrin having caused an allergic rash, I received a nebuliser dose every month for a year; and just when that stopped (and they were pretty sure that I wouldn't be needing *more* blood) about two thirds of a pint of blood was now *removed* and gallingly (for an ex-blood donor) thrown in the bin – again every month for a year. You see, through having received up to 30 pints of blood, I'd ended up with the iron of over 12 men! Now willing again to look up conditions on the internet, I found that an iron overdose causes a number of symptoms. As the first was *death*, I didn't bother to look at the others.

Life was full of these amazing facts – I could surprise folk by telling them my blood group was now O positive, rather than my AB negative – as the donor could only make *his own* blood type (although I'd enjoyed belonging to 'a rare blood group', pride really). I learned I had at least 5 infections in hospital and their names. One day I tried to draw my Consultant out and asked: 'Why did I have to stay in hospital for 5 months for chemo when other cancer patients go in as a day patient, or else have it by tablet at home . . . was mine *10 times* stronger?' I put that forward as a ridiculous number, thinking she'd say *it was* 2 or 3 times, instead of which she answered, 'more like *a 100*'. (I'm guessing that's why the 'cold cap' helmet was a non-starter.)

I even managed to get *a job* . . . as carer for my parents (shared with my sister Jayne). It was hard at times as Dad had dementia and could wake at 3.30 thinking it was morning! He passed away 4 months before this *final* email I sent around, while sharing Mum's care with my sister.

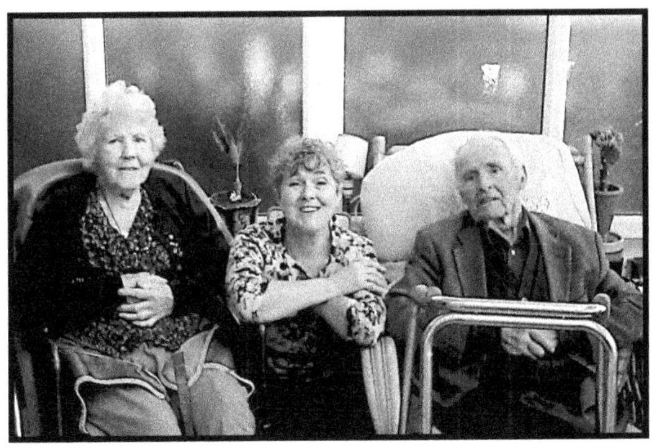

Final Dispatch

Dear All,

Today 12th January 2020 marks a special day for me. On this date in 2015, after the 2nd round of chemo, my Leukaemia was declared to be 'in remission' (all clear).

5 years of remission = CURED! according to the medical profession.

This morning I thanked my church for their prayers and went for a meal with two friends.

Be glad with me!

And thanks for your support/prayers.

Hazel

War Correspondent turns Author

Somehow I managed not to have noticed the passing of the 6th anniversary last month. I think that is healthy.

Composing those dispatches wasn't hard – I was in general quite interested in the world I'd somehow arrived in. Where else can you chat to a woman opposite who is on arsenic, and a man in the day room on thalidomide? I was on a cocktail of 3 brands of chemo. What's your poison? It seemed to me perhaps any poison would do!

Writing the emails also gave me some satisfaction – along with directing from my hospital bed, the small trickle of work arriving into my business, to various dancers & drummers. They were both reasons, besides sock washing, to force my way up out of chemo lethargy. And I do enjoy my own jokes created therein ('*gallows humor*' as my friend from New York termed it!) Who first said laughter is good medicine? I wouldn't make a comedian however, due to the disadvantage of many not even realising I'm making jokes! Nevertheless, if I *want* folk to laugh, I can *sing*, that seems to work – it's that farcical face that occurs! (Nobody laughs when I *dance*, I must add to preserve a modicum of dignity!) Those who know who they are, can afford to laugh at themselves: Bob Monkhouse's line, 'When I told folk I was going to be a comedian, they all *laughed*: well! – they're not laughing *now*!'

But anyhow my role as *war correspondent*, I am laying firmly aside, by sending these dispatches on for publication as I finally found a young person who knew how to!

He asked me '*what I had learnt*' through it all, well – apart from a lot of medical jargon, and that nurses & doctors are far more interested in their patients than in each other (my previous impression from TV dramas) – I guess to increase that 'ability to dwell in uncertainty', which gave me an advantage in the later Covid crisis, over others whose lives were impoverished by predictability.

Home from hospital, feeling precarious, there were nights when I went to bed and wondered whether I'd be alive in the morning. The question wouldn't keep me awake. On rousing I'd say to myself, as a point of information, '*Oh . . . I am alive*'.

Christmas 1939 with all the uncertainties George VI quoted these words:

And I said to the man
who stood at the gate of the year:
"Give me a light
that I may tread safely into the unknown."
And he replied:
"*Go out* into the darkness
and put your hand into the Hand of God.
That shall be to you better than light
and safer than a known way."

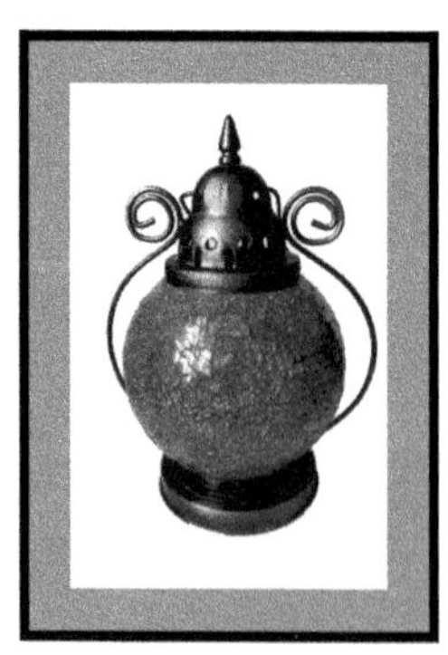

Take it from an Old Soldier

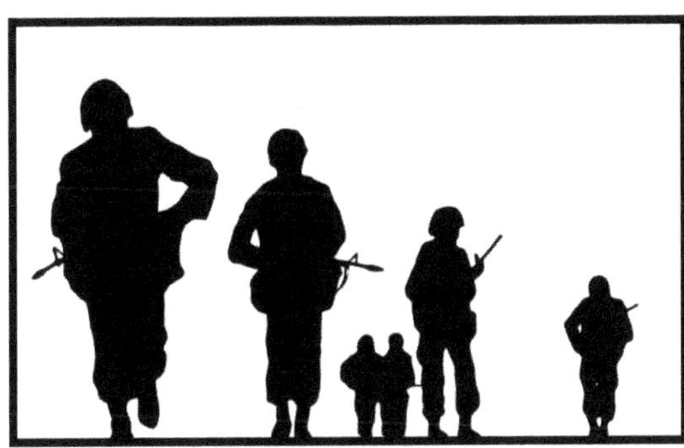

Another thing I learnt, was how to be a better hospital visitor myself, and about mistakes I must have made in the past. Don't get me wrong, I enjoyed most visits. During the visits of various church friends there was a quiet prayer for me. But folk, don't pray *too loud* in an open ward – it's kind of embarrassing when you leave!

Some visitors stayed too long. I think of the friend for whom I was a captive audience: I was the patient on the bed, but she was the patient on the couch, and fell into long monologues about her childhood (in such circumstances, perhaps it is not rude to 'fall asleep'.)

Others talked nervously without stop. Mates – Leukaemia is *tiring*, chemo *exhausting* and trying to follow constant flitting from topic to topic *saps* the little bit of energy you've got! Remember Job's 'comforters' giving him great support for that first 7 days by sitting with him in the dust in silence. The problem began after that when they started to speak!

Male visitors generally did better at this – although the opening line I had from one, of *how long have the doctors given you*? is probably best avoided!

On the other hand, an *interactive* conversation may be life enhancing – I had a discussion with one of the drummers on the simsimiyya (an Egyptian harp) and its use in Port Said. Absolutely amazing! It didn't remind me of who I'd been, it reminded me of who I still was.

I was grateful to those who braved their fear of hospitals, but there were those who didn't come; conspicuous by their absence. Months later, I asked Gurmiet (who had first come on that mercy mission with left-over curry and not been seen since) why? She said she *had* come to Barts to visit accompanied by her daughter, but had not been able to actually face coming upstairs . . . to see me *just lying there*, instead of my usual lively self. Not visiting may not equal not caring.

On the patient's side, I was actually interested in my visitors' news, and hopefully didn't start talking about myself before they even asked. After all, they represent the outside world and it's good to have contact with it – especially if they can bring in food that doesn't smell, such as salad, for the bedside fridge Barts supplies – ooh ah! (That is unless in the period when the microbes on raw food are too dangerous to risk.) For by 11.30 I could start dreading the arrival of the food trolley and the impending nausea!

If I was giving advice from 'When I WAS in the *WAR*', I'd say a few things, such as *ask for a blood test* earlier than I had one if health is breaking down (failure to heal small things etc), or even with just a strange tiredness. Mentioning tiredness to *friends* brought the response, 'Oh *I* feel tired *too*!' Mention it to a *doctor* and *ask*, before you end up in A&E (some never know they have Leukaemia, it's just on their death certificate.) When I went back to my GP (who'd given me 4 prescriptions with the advice to come back in 2 weeks if not better) to tell him what had actually been wrong with me, I lifted my wig and said 'Leukaemia'. He replied that it is hard to diagnose. Perhaps the problem is more that it's hard to suspect.

I wouldn't even have gone to A&E that October day if I'd had the option of staying home in bed, with someone to bring me cups of tea and cheese on toast! Once in Barts, I asked the doctor what would have happened if I hadn't gone. 'Well', he replied, 'by Christmas you would have had a major infection, which we *might* have been able to cure, but which may have left you *too weak* for chemo.'

Also, when in hospital *don't be afraid to speak up*. Express your concerns politely, but firmly. Possibly the time I was in most danger was when – between chemos with little resistance to any infection – due to a temperature I spent the week on a *general* ward in the *local* hospital. The child visiting his Gran in the bed so close coughed away, while his father commented that it was good his cough was coming out! To the doctor's question as to how I felt, I replied 'I feel like I'm sleeping on the edge of hell and trying not to roll in!' Shortly afterwards I was given a side room. My dramatic response was effective! My concern however *was* justifiable – I didn't want to die unnecessarily – but my belief is that it was *heaven* I would roll up at! As the Calypso song goes, 'Everybody wants to go to heaven, but nobody wants to die!'

My natural drama didn't always work: one time, when an outpatient, the hospital doctor was assessing whether or not to take me back in again. It was a freezing cold day, and I conveyed exactly how I felt with: 'I wouldn't care if you said you'd throw me out the window; I'd just turn up my collar and lie on the pavement'. He sent me home.

And a suggestion for us all: whenever you see anyone you care about under great stress, *lavish your time on them then* (if they'd like that, and you are able) – *without telling them what to do* (unless they ask.) There may not be this need later; who knows, if sickness is a possibility, you may help them avoid it! Rogue cells are constantly occurring in every one of us, but not sleeping can lower the immune system; that's when the errant cells, spy-like, go undetected.

But if there *is* a hit, that's the time to *pull out the stops*. St Paul's stands out amongst the rubble in that Blitz picture – but it is not the case that miraculously it avoided getting hit; rather that the fire fighters and wardens were focused on saving it. Churchill's orders of course (by every effort that national symbol had to stand.) I think of when I had the rigours and my body shuddered. *I don't know what's happening to me* I thought *but I'm not sure my heart can take it* – for it was squeezed as tight as a clam. Feeling cold in my fever, I had foolishly piled my coat etc. on my bed exacerbating it – but fortunately I was in a specialist hospital, and the nurses both knew what to do, and also were intent on my survival. As for the 'dedicated nurse' I had decided to stick with, she did indeed prove 'awfully good at her job'!

Recipients of the email dispatches were also standing by holding the hosepipes, doing *whatever* they could. A hamper, visits, offers of books, a West African talisman, cards, the prayers of Muslims and Bible verses from Christians – I recognised all as acts stemming from the urge to help on the part of the particular givers.

When recovering, *take encouragement* from whatever possible: for me, it was being steady enough on my feet not to have dogs bark at me, or drunks in the street thinking I was *one of them*; walking half way round a field – eventually all the way round – and the day coming when the bandaged port in the arm concealing the tubes was finally removed making showering no longer hazardous. Imagine the boost for me, when I was able to say '*I'll do it*!' to cover a school workshop, when the dancer assigned was ill!

Lastly, never forget *you are not the only one* to be bombed, everyone has their troubles, including those who come to visit. Remember too that *others have survived*. On leaving hospital after the transplant, in chatting to the cab driver, he shared that his young daughter had had a stem cell transplant. Coincidence? I hardly spoke to anyone new outside of a hospital, but here again besides the bank girl on the phone, was contact with someone who'd survived a transplant!

The Elephant on the Battlefield

Some musings on the unmentioned but perhaps not unthought: the email 'Friends 23' & the 2 subsequent ones, tossed around ideas on why bad things like illness happen – *but why did I survive*?

Why do some and not others?

They are also prized. God's love is toward, and not against, everyone. The 'nasty patient' survived too – I came across her in outpatients sometime later, and she was no spring chick either.

I only read the blog of one other person with AML when I was in hospital, the young Jewish New Yorker in a university hospital. He expected to survive because he was young. He had every reason to expect that. The odds were in his favour.

He didn't make it. Why did I with the odds stacked against me age-wise, and a chromosome change in the Leukaemia cells in the 3rd and worst category? (Although not *the worst of the worst* category as the doctor said being cheery.) I guess the easy answer is that someone has to be in the minority in his group who die; and that someone has to be in the minority in my group who live.

Naturally that answer satisfies no one who is in the frame. 'Why me?' has been asked since time immemorial (no one it seems asks 'Why *not* me?')

One can point to factors such as underlying health (the doctors were pleased I wasn't a smoker and was physically active), and to the proficiency of the hospital – not just the professionalism of the medics, but also the professionalism of the cleaners zapping those germs! I was privileged to be in St Bartholomew's under a National Health Service, but there are no guarantees in the best hospitals. Access to medical treatment worldwide is patently unfair and that is something to be angry about, but there is no certainty *of life*, or else *of death*, whatever hospital you are in.

However, ultimately our question why some and not others, is going to be unanswerable – and not everyone can cope with that. Myself, I was philosophical about dying, although I had a preference to live, and simply put myself in God's hands for the whatever. I had no word from above that I would make it but dared to take encouragement from God-incidences. On the other hand, I'd known Christians with more faith than myself, who fully believed that they'd survive. But they didn't.

Largely however, my faith is in God, not in what he will *do* for me. I believe I came near the brink, particularly in the *rigours*, and the lack of specialist care in the *local* hospital. I would have accepted either outcome, but I do *thank* God I came through.

I absolutely love the story of the 3 Jewish men in Babylon who wouldn't bow down to the King's golden idol. He threatens to throw them into a fiery furnace and asks: '*Then what God* will be able to rescue you from my hand?' They answer his question in 3 parts: firstly that *there is* a God who can rescue them; secondly that *he will*; and thirdly, my favourite bit, that *even if he doesn't* they're not going to worship his idol *anyway*! Awkward beggars? Or men with the same lack of priority for outcome?

(The ending is superfluous to my point, but they are

seen walking in the fire with a 4th man 'who looks like a son of the gods', and survive.)

After initially being admitted to Barts unexpectedly, friends brought nightdresses. One held up, was long and white with laced cotton. I was in genuine admiration – but not for *immediate* needs: 'Oh! That would make a *lovely* shroud!' I exclaimed. It wasn't exactly what my friend wanted to hear. (I have kept it by since, all *any* of us have is time.)

Does prayer alter the stakes? I think it can. However, I myself didn't pray for me – I could no more be a 'prayer warrior' at that time than enter a boxing ring. Others prayed for me – including one I was told who got angry with cancer & prayed with verve!

I can never repay all that was done for me, not only in this and other ways, but also in terms of the cost to the NHS. I hope Barts will forgive me if my perceptions at any point are incorrect; and also 'recollections may vary'.

Now these emails are available to a wider audience, it remains for me to wish all the very best to you Readers, whoever & wherever you are!

And if you are similarly diagnosed, think of Terri who stayed on the regular chemo and didn't even need a stem cell transplant, or else remember the Prof's words 'It is possible to have a cure'.

God bless,

Hazel

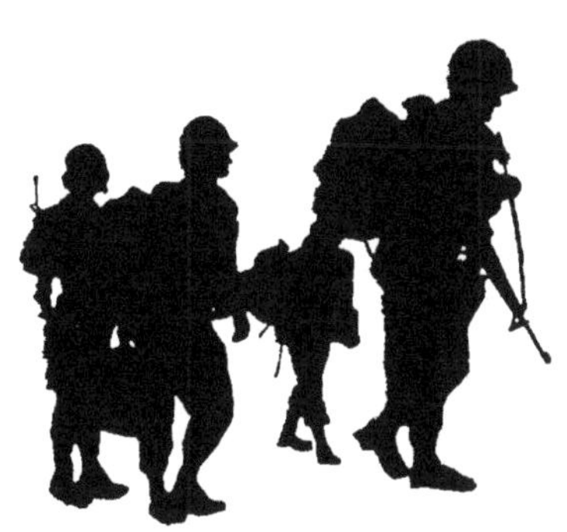

Home to barracks.
Thanks guys!

Photo Credits

1. Cover photo – Miles Mooney. (Miles also sat with me through the transplant.)
2. Author Shot – Victoria Jenkins (my niece).
3. 'Publicity Shot' for school workshops – Tim Garside. (Tim was also the Master Drummer.)
4. 1916 fun sketch – *The Graphic* (1916).
5. St. Bartholomew's Hospital (showing St. Paul's) – Barts Health NHS Trust.
6. World War II ceramic poppies – Ron Ellis/ Shutterstock.com.
7. Soldier with gun – UK Ministry of Defence.
8. Strictly photo by friend and fellow fan – Kathy Hester.
9. Fireworks display at St. Paul's Cathedral – Pajor Pawel/ Shutterstock.com.
10. Lord Mayor's Show – www.citymatters.london.
11. Troops of the 1st Australian Division in Belgium, WWI – National Library of Australia.
12. Homerton Hospital – Courtesy of Michael G. Spafford.
13. St. Paul's in the snow – r/london Reddit community.
14. St. Paul's in the Blitz – Imperial War Museums.
15. Rescue by the Americans – US Marine Corps.
16. Rescue by the Russians – Reuters.
17. The giant leap – Shutterstock.com.
18. Bart Simpson – Shutterstock.com.
19. London Marathon – Nicola Pfund (www.nicolapfund.ch).
20. The colonial officer – www.gentlemansgazette.com.
21. Bear – Courtesy of Loren Mooney.
22. St. Bartholomew's Hospital 1702 gate – www.microsoft.localdataimages.com.
23. Zanzibar Festival – Sauti Za Busara official Flickr page.
24. Back cover photo – John Connor, CEO.
25. Selfies & hospital indoor shots – Hazel.

www.ingramcontent.com/pod-product-compliance
Ingram Content Group UK Ltd.
Pitfield, Milton Keynes, MK11 3LW, UK
UKHW020140250726
13967UKWH00002B/775